DAVID KIRSCH'S

Ultimate Family Wellness

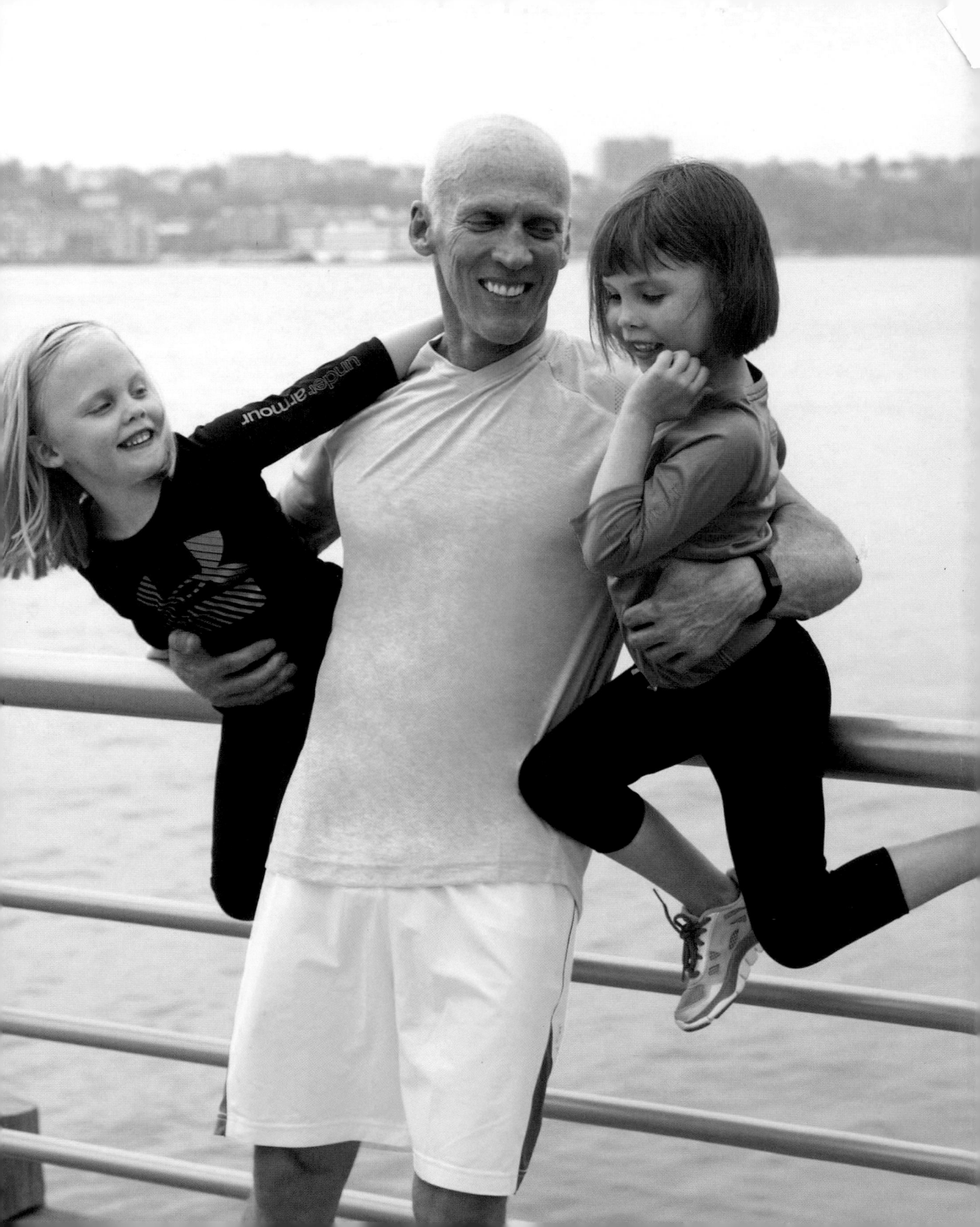

DAVID KIRSCH'S

Ultimate Family Wellness

The No-Excuses Program for Diet, Fitness, and Lifelong Health

DAVID KIRSCH

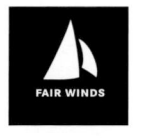

FAIR WINDS

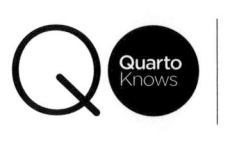

Quarto is the authority on a wide range of topics.

Quarto educates, entertains and enriches the lives of our readers—enthusiasts and lovers of hands-on living.

www.QuartoKnows.com

First published in the United States of America in 2016 by

Fair Winds Press, an imprint of

Quarto Publishing Group USA Inc.

100 Cummings Center

Suite 406-L

Beverly, Massachusetts 01915-6101

Telephone: (978) 282-9590

Fax: (978) 283-2742

QuartoKnows.com

Visit our blogs at QuartoKnows.com

20 19 18 17 16   1 2 3 4 5

ISBN: 978-1-59233-709-5

Digital edition published in 2016
eISBN: 978-1-62788-837-0

Library of Congress Cataloging-in-Publication Data available

Cover Image: Luciana Pampalone
Cover Design: Quarto Publishing Group USA
Book Design and Layout: Sporto
Photography: Luciana Pampalone, except pages 12, 108–111 (various), 122, 211, and 216 courtesy of David Kirsch; and pages 130–132 shutterstock.com

Printed in China

The information in this book is for educational purposes only. It is not intended to replace the advice of a physician or medical practitioner. Please see your health-care provider before beginning any new health program.

Emilia & Francesca

You are my heart and soul.

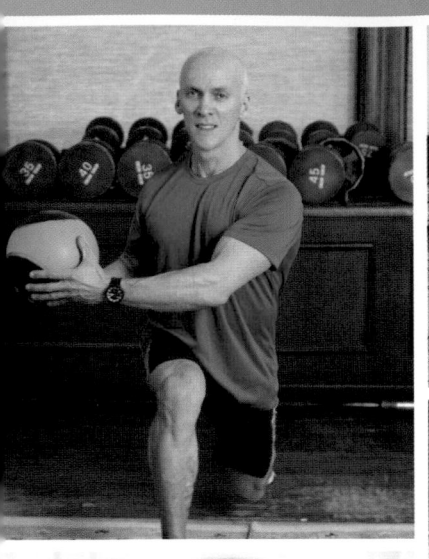
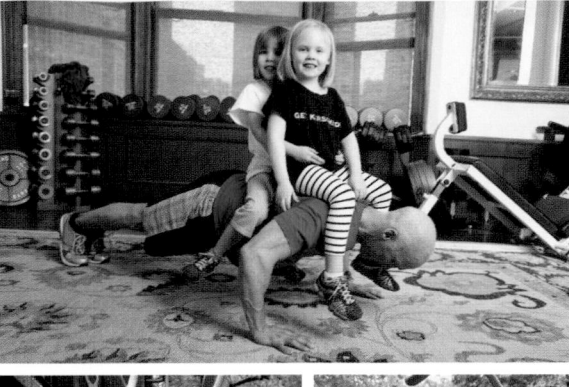
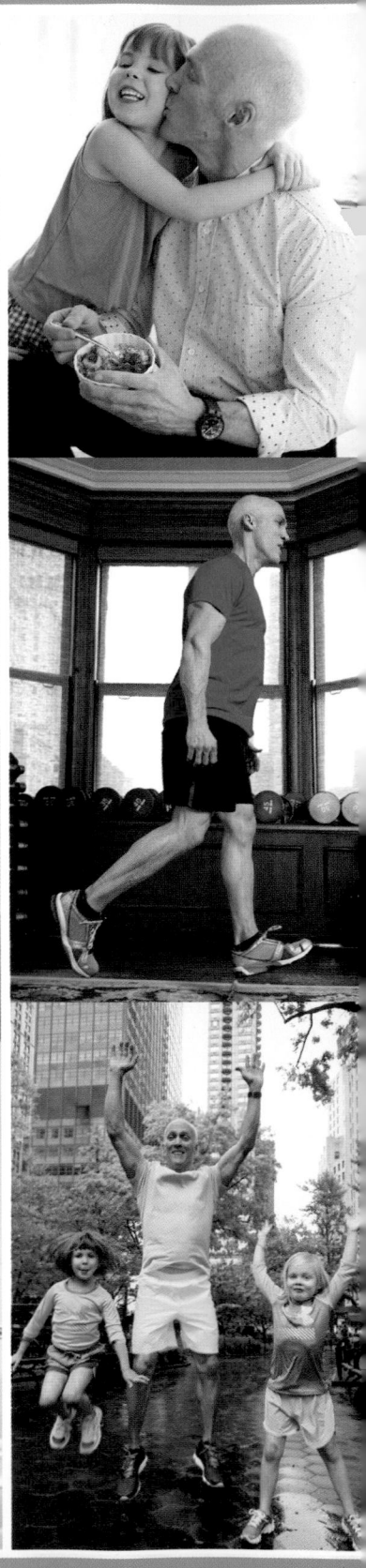
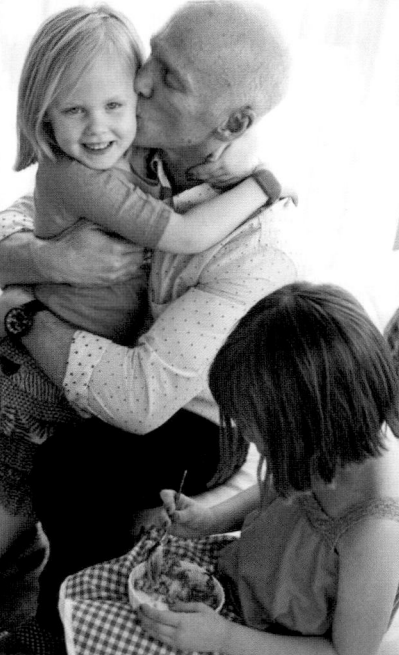
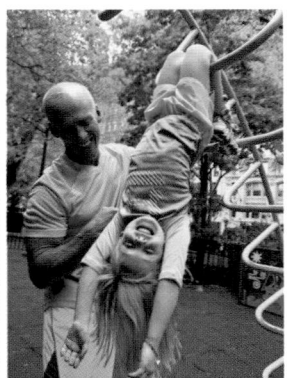
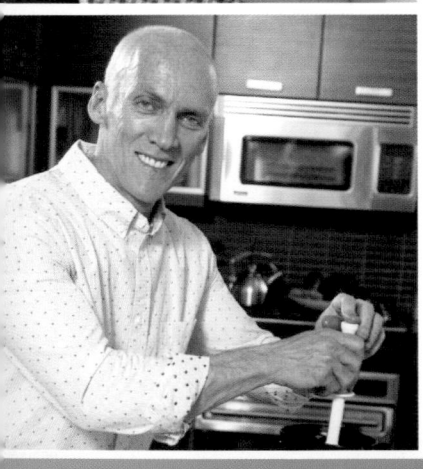
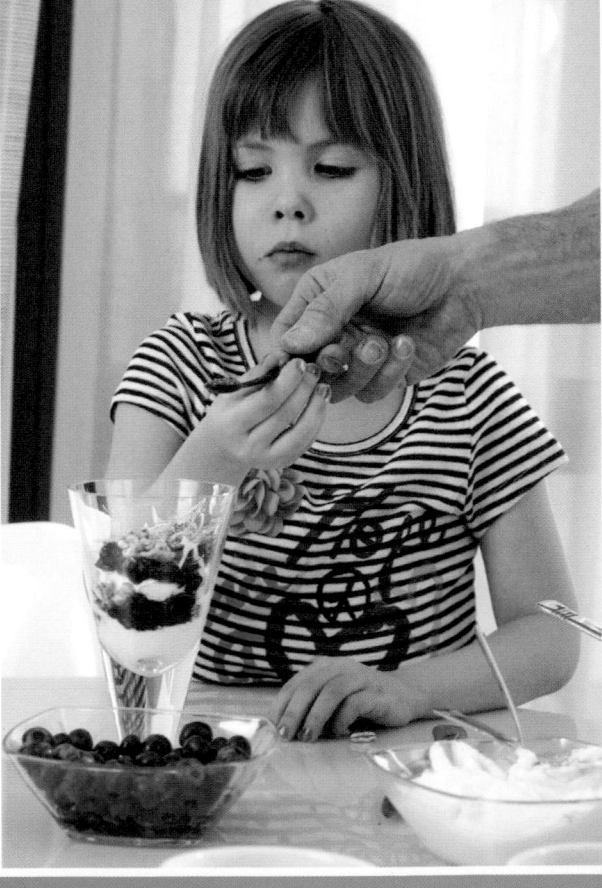

CONTENTS

Foreword by Jennifer Lopez   8

Introduction   11

CHAPTER 1

What Is the 5-5-5 Program® and the Ultimate Family Wellness Plan?   21

CHAPTER 2

Exercising and Activities   29

CHAPTER 3

Nutrition, Food, and Family   113

CHAPTER 4

Cooking with Your Kids   141

CHAPTER 5

Management and Maintenance Made Easy   201

Acknowledgments   214

About the Author   216

Resources   217

Index   222

FOREWORD

When I was asked to write the foreword to this book, *David Kirsch's Ultimate Family Wellness*, I thought to myself: What is it about this book that makes it so special—that sets it apart from so many of the other fitness books out there?

First, like David, I am a busy working parent of twins. I was immediately drawn to the title. Who amongst us doesn't want to be The Ultimate Wellness Family? From really delicious, easy-to-prepare five-ingredient recipes that Max, Emme, and I can make to beautiful moments of movement together on our bikes, scooters, or in the playground, David's message is very real, accessible, and timely. We live in a world that is so fast-paced and frenetic that we often don't find time to "organically" connect with our family. Second, I thought, what is it about David that makes him so special and unique? Surely I have worked with many good trainers, but David's approach to fitness is unique. From our first meeting, I felt at ease. He was able to customize a workout for my body and goals. I love that he is able to change-up the workouts, always keep my body guessing, and always leave me feeling Kirsched!

We are both born and bred New Yorkers, and I had a sense that he knew me, knew my body, and knew exactly what to do to energize me and help me realize my best self! Like him, I wear many hats—businesswoman, entrepreneur, and, most important, mother of twins!

David's story is such a beautiful one. After years of being one of the most sought out trainers in the world, he decided he wanted to become a single parent. Little did he know that his dream would multiply by two! Although I haven't had the opportunity to spend much time with David, Emilia, and Francesca, I have had the pleasure of meeting them at the Madison Square Club. I have watched how loving and tender he is with them and the joy in his eyes when he speaks about them. I thought, here's a guy that gets it. Although he is devoted to his business and his many clients, his family is his first priority. Throughout the book, the photographs of David, Emilia, and Francesca cooking, exercising, and just having fun send a powerful message to parents everywhere; Good health and family wellness is easily accessible for all. I recommend this book for anyone, who, like me, wants the Ultimate Wellness Family. The time is now!

-Jennifer Lopez

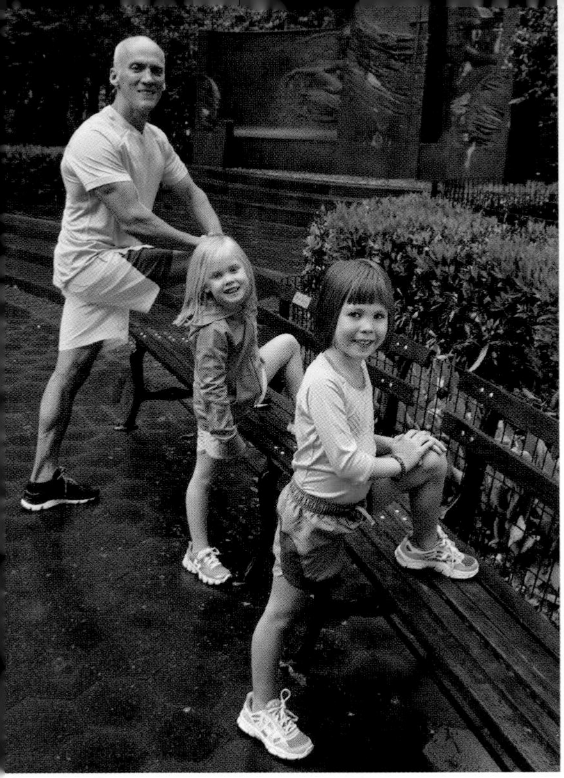

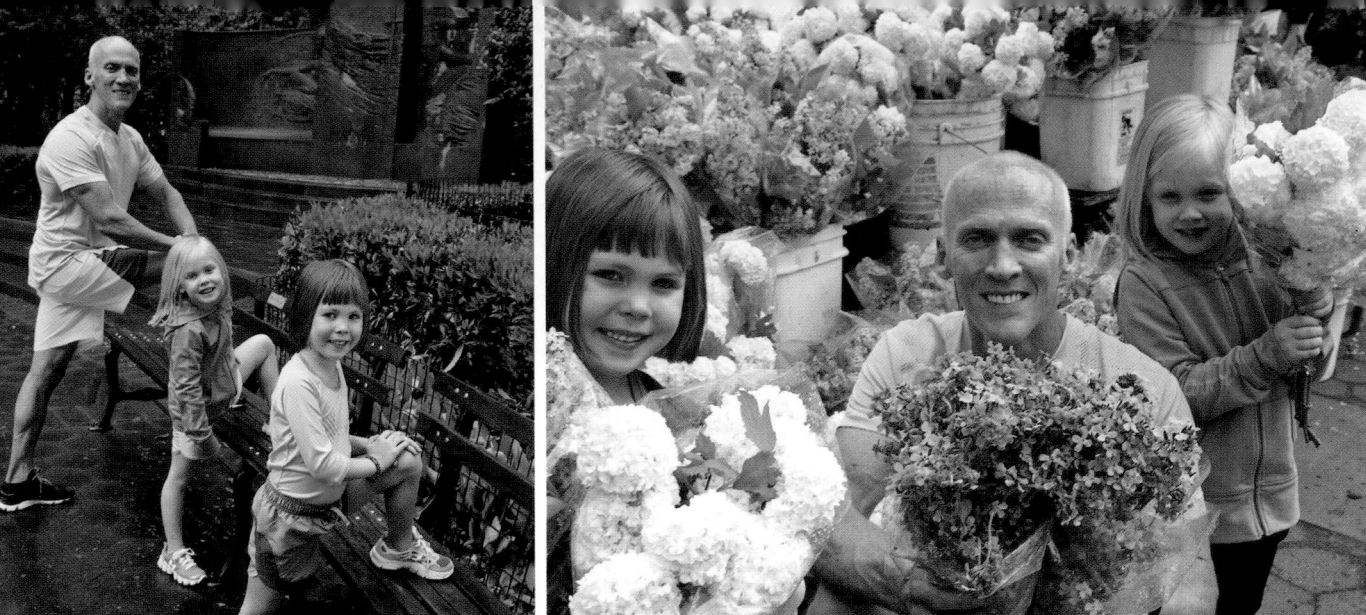

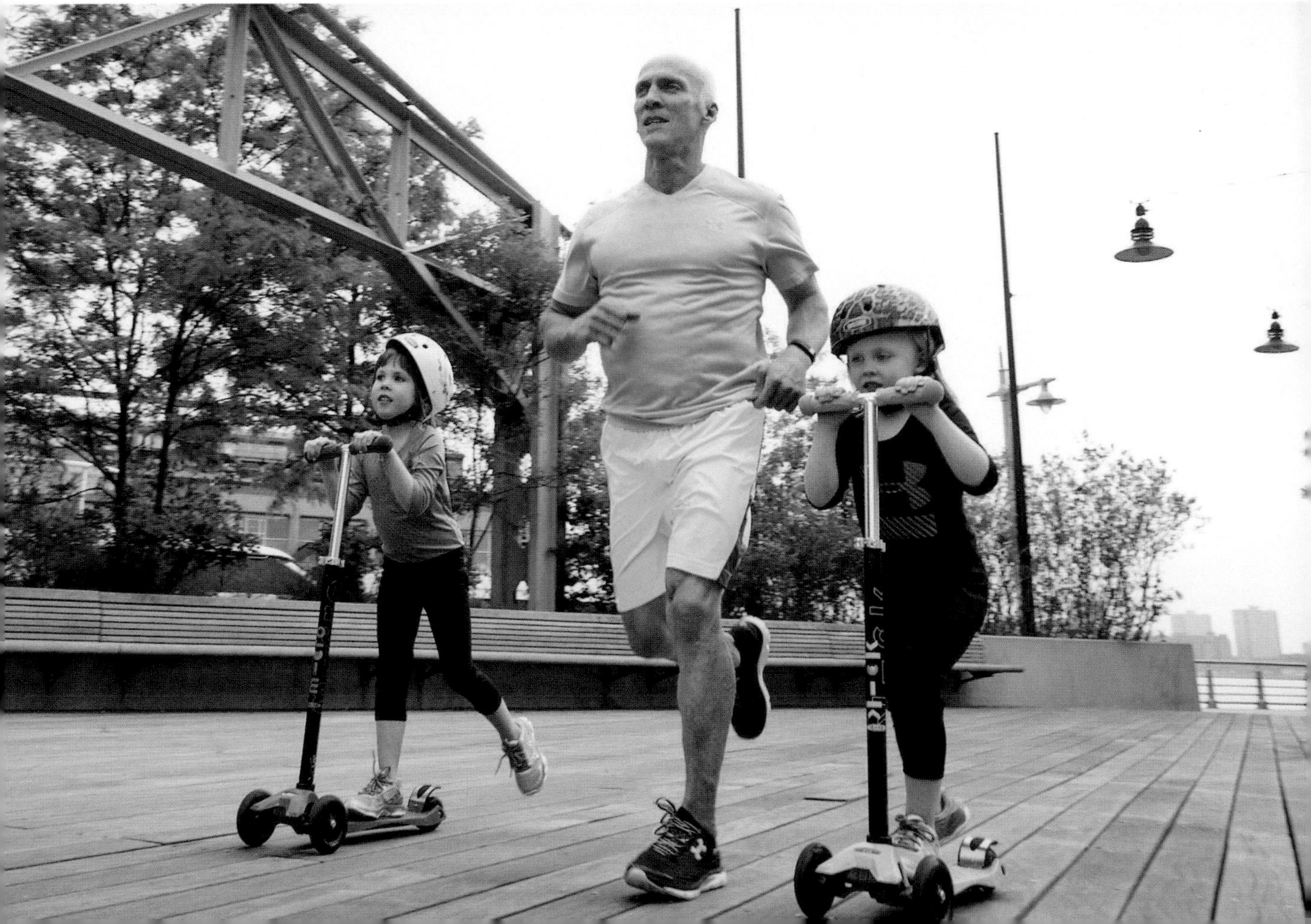

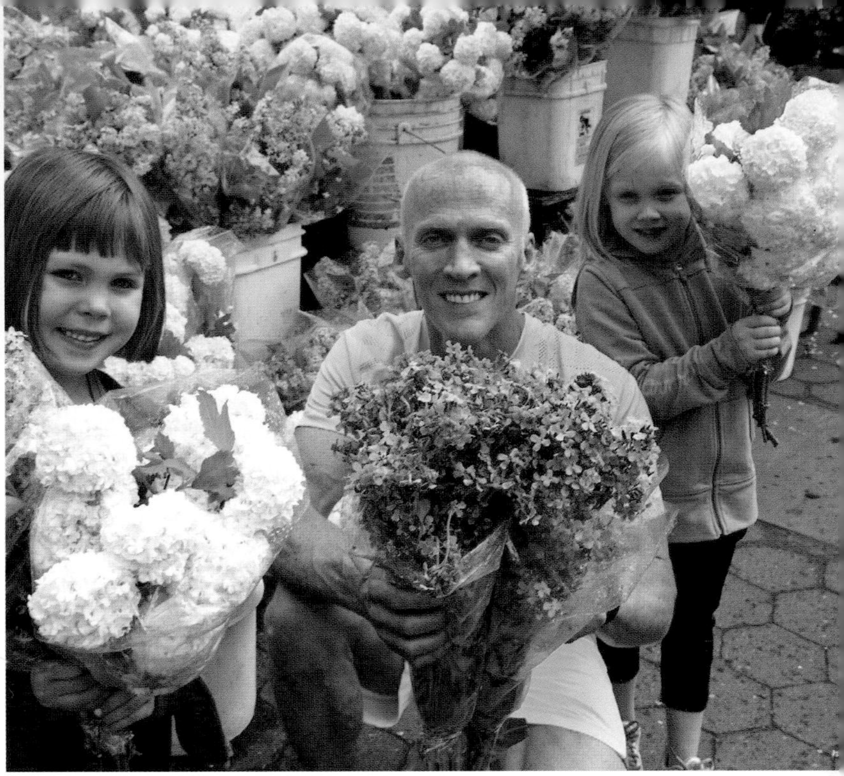

INTRODUCTION

In the twenty-five years that I have been part of the fitness industry, I have watched many trends come and go. Since my last book, *The Ultimate New York Diet*, the publishing world has dramatically changed. Social media has exploded and anything you want to know is readily available via the Internet. In addition to YouTube, Facebook, Twitter, Instagram, and Pinterest, a plethora of fitness, nutrition, and weight-loss apps are available in your back pocket or purse. Weight-loss programs such as *The Biggest Loser* and "self-help" shows such as *Dr. Oz* are a remote click away any time of day.

So with all of this information literally at your fingertips, I ask myself, "Why write another book?" What can I say? Is there any wisdom or information I can impart that isn't readily available? What unique fitness viewpoint can I offer without radically departing from the core beliefs and tenets I set forth in my first book, *Sound Mind, Sound Body*?

Then I realized that the myriad resources out there addressing weight loss, body transformation, and diets from fasting to juicing put us on information overload. It is very confusing. What I offer is a single voice, from a single parent, to give you a simple, easy-to-follow wellness guide for you and your family. To me, fitness has become so much more than looking good on the beach or losing those final five (or ten) pounds. *Wellness* has become the lexicon for everything healthy as it transcends fitness to include living a healthy lifestyle, raising a healthy family, and learning about nutrition. Don't get me wrong, I love training Kate Upton, Jennifer Lopez, and Liv Tyler (a few of the celebrity clients who I work with and consider friends). I am grateful for what they and other past clients have contributed to my success. Although I am proudly still known as the "Master of the Ass®" and the Body Sculptor™, I am equally proud to be known as a fitness, lifestyle, and wellness expert—and most proud to be a father!

REWRITING MY STORY

One of the unique things about my previous books was the inclusion of my personal anecdotes and those of my clients' inspiring journeys. I've always felt I'd rather tell a relatable story—whether mine or a client's—than give a lecture. What's changed in my life and the world of fitness in the eight years since I wrote and published my most recent book? The answer is, quite simply, plenty.

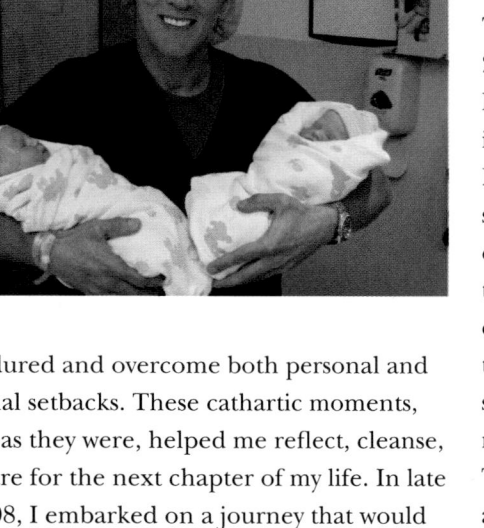

I have endured and overcome both personal and professional setbacks. These cathartic moments, as painful as they were, helped me reflect, cleanse, and prepare for the next chapter of my life. In late spring 2008, I embarked on a journey that would forever change me.

I had always wanted to be a father, but having devoted my entire adult life to my career, I saw little time or opportunity to realize that dream. When the right time came, I did what I always do when I have a goal in mind: I set out with steely-eyed determination on my path. Being a person who loosely believes in the general characteristics of the zodiac, I've had my astrological chart done and found that as a Capricorn, I tend to be logical, focused, and highly driven while also being emotional, loving, and nurturing. I have been able to successfully employ all of these characteristics

in my professional life as a trainer and I felt it also prepared me for the next and most important phase of my life—becoming a father.

That process started in 2008, and on August 25, 2009, Emilia and Francesca were born in Sioux Falls, South Dakota, with my mother at my side in the delivery room. My gestational carrier, Michelle, delivered my two angels. Emilia weighed seven pounds, two ounces, Francesca, six pounds, eight ounces. Michelle remains a part of our lives today. I'll never forget the feeling of holding my daughters for the first time. My guardian angels— the people no longer here with me, but I know, spiritually, are omnipresent—helped me realize my greatest dream. I held new life in my arms. Their birth strengthened and enriched my life and gave me new purpose. Being a loving, single father brings me more joy and happiness than I ever before realized. And lessons I have learned as a single parent have helped me evolve as a fitness and wellness professional, too. *Healthy l iving* and *healthy eating* are not just "hashtag" phrases; they are a regular part of my life and my daughters' lives.

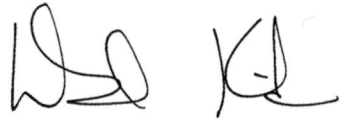

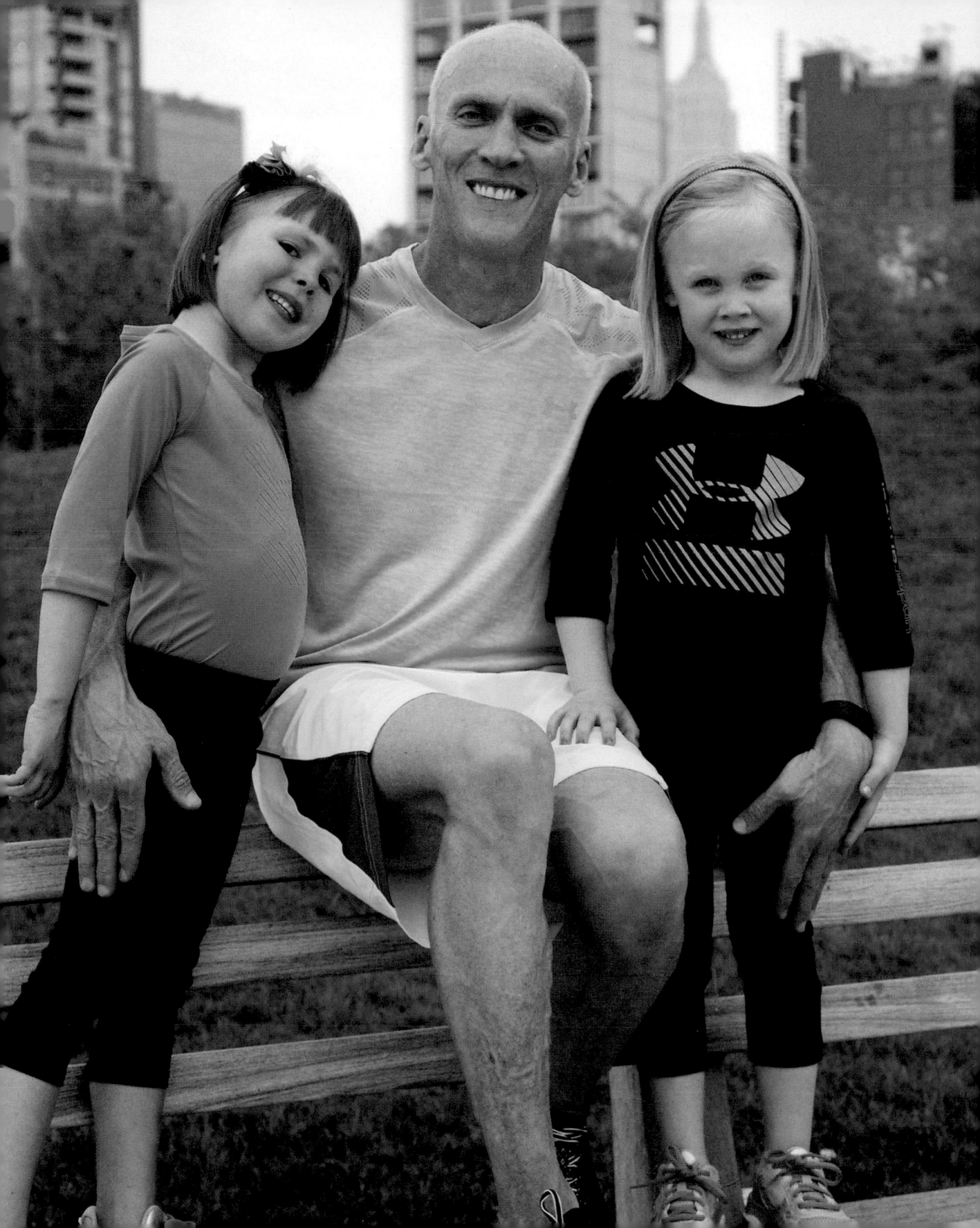

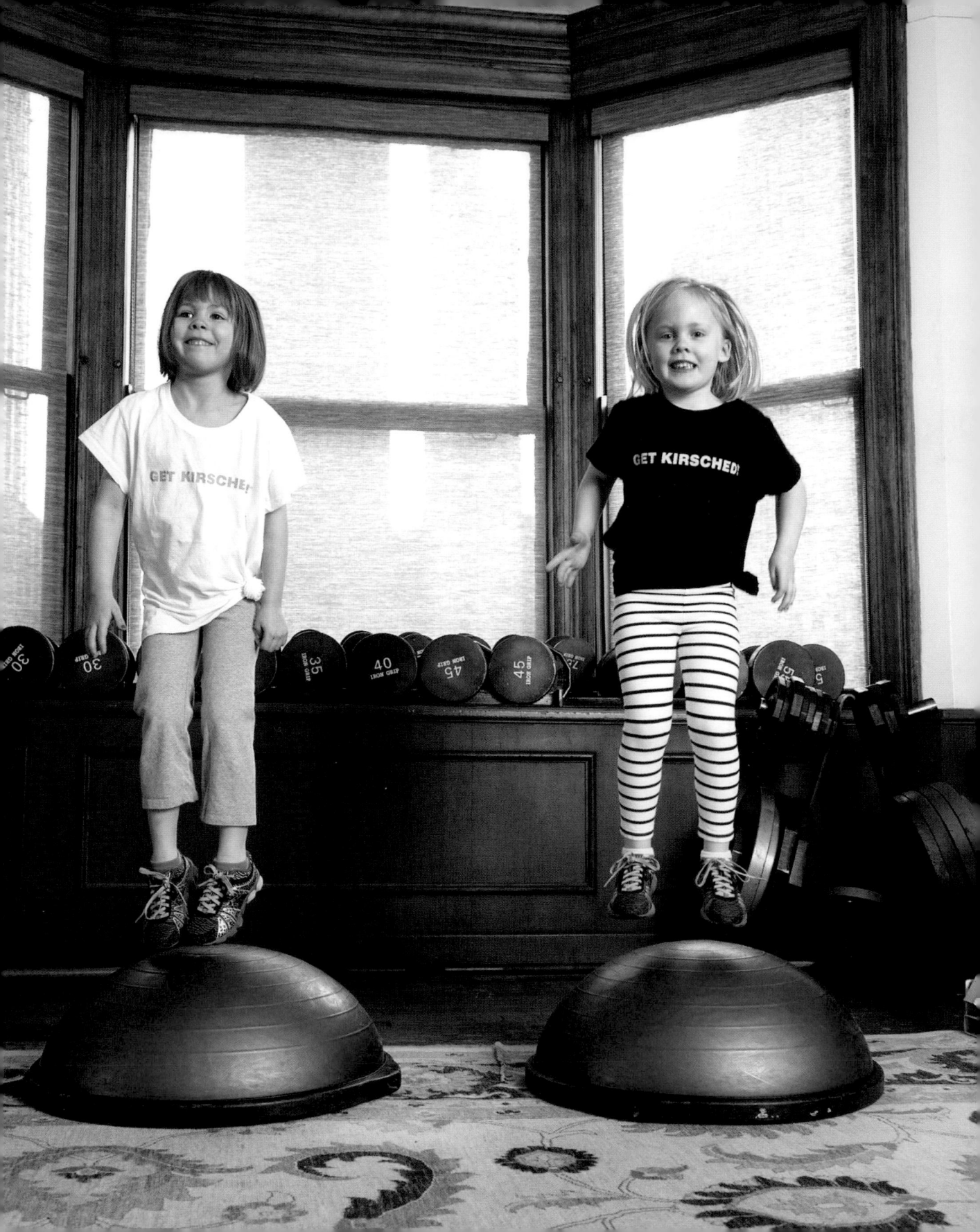

NEW PRIORITIES REQUIRE A REFOCUS

Although being a parent hasn't changed how I feel about living a healthful, balanced life, I am a gentler, kinder, more inclusive fitness/wellness expert. I have learned to accept that I am far from perfect; that like life itself, wellness isn't black or white. You might say the girls added color to my life. My priorities have changed, and I don't always have ninety minutes for a workout like I did before they were born. I have been forced (through home and work responsibilities) to modify my workouts and loosen my—and my family's—dietary restrictions. Although we don't always eat perfectly healthy meals, I try to make the best choices from the foods available.

Whenever you experience a significant change in your life—a new job, a move, a relationship, the birth of a child—your focus changes. The Ultimate Family Wellness Plan was born soon after Emilia and Francesca, and it developed out of necessity. Sleepless nights, challenges at work, and carving out "me time" are increasingly difficult. Quite simply, as a single father, I needed to get my workouts "on the fly." In a sense, the more "hats" I wore (single parent, business entrepreneur, and author), the more I needed something to keep me grounded. More than ever, I could relate to my clients and their demanding schedules—the never-ending balancing act that is life. I think about calls I have gotten from clients about being stuck at the office, being called out of state on a last-minute trip, or the most recent one—the nanny called in sick and I am stuck at home with the kids.

It is 8 p.m. on a Sunday night and I have just put the girls to sleep. It was a very full weekend, and a trip to the gym wasn't on the agenda. For my sanity, and to reconnect my brain to my body, I just completed two sets of fifty pushups.

The Ultimate Family Wellness Plan is all about finding time—wherever, whenever—to engage your mind and body. Never one to play victim, I sat down one night and started developing the concept for what would become the program in this book. It quickly turned into much more than a weight-loss and fitness plan. Sure, there is a real promise: 5 minutes plus 5 days (5 exercises) equals 5 pounds of weight loss. But its accessibility and ease of use—who doesn't have five minutes a day?—make it a program you can easily integrate into your family life. In fact, 5-5-5 is the perfect way to jump-start your wellness program.

The program is a total lifestyle transformation and guide. Gone are the myriad excuses for not embracing a healthier lifestyle for you and your family. It is accessible, affordable, and "excuse-proof." It has changed Emilia's, Francesca's, and my life immeasurably. We are an Ultimate Wellness Family!

YOUR FAMILY'S NEW WELLNESS PLAN

The 5-5-5 Program® is a short-term weight-loss and toning program for you (see chapter 5), and after those initial five days, there is an exceedingly achievable long-term nutrition and fitness plan I'm calling the Ultimate Family Wellness Plan. Once you successfully complete the 5-5-5 Program, you'll see how its principles—short bursts of exercise (activity) and quick and healthy ways to prepare meals—are easy to apply to your everyday family life. These principles are the essence of what makes up the Ultimate Family Wellness Plan, making it a program for all, and for all time.

Believe me when I say that some exercise is better than none. A short, intense exercise circuit of five minutes can work more effectively than a sixty-minute unfocused workout because it connects mind and body, making you mentally more alert and energized. And once you successfully complete the plan, you'll see how easily and naturally its tenets integrate into your everyday lifestyle. In this way, the plan can help you realize your fitness goals in a short time, resulting in positive feelings of success and motivating you to incorporate some, if not all, aspects of the program into long-term lifestyle changes.

The book is divided into sections on fitness, nutrition, recipes, and maintenance and lifestyle.

Personal Fitness, Family Activities

The exercise portion of this book focuses on effective exercises. Although the 5-5-5 Program was initially designed to jump-start a fit and healthy lifestyle that has you losing five pounds in just five days, it has evolved into so much more. It is a highly customizable program that you can adapt for your specific body type to help

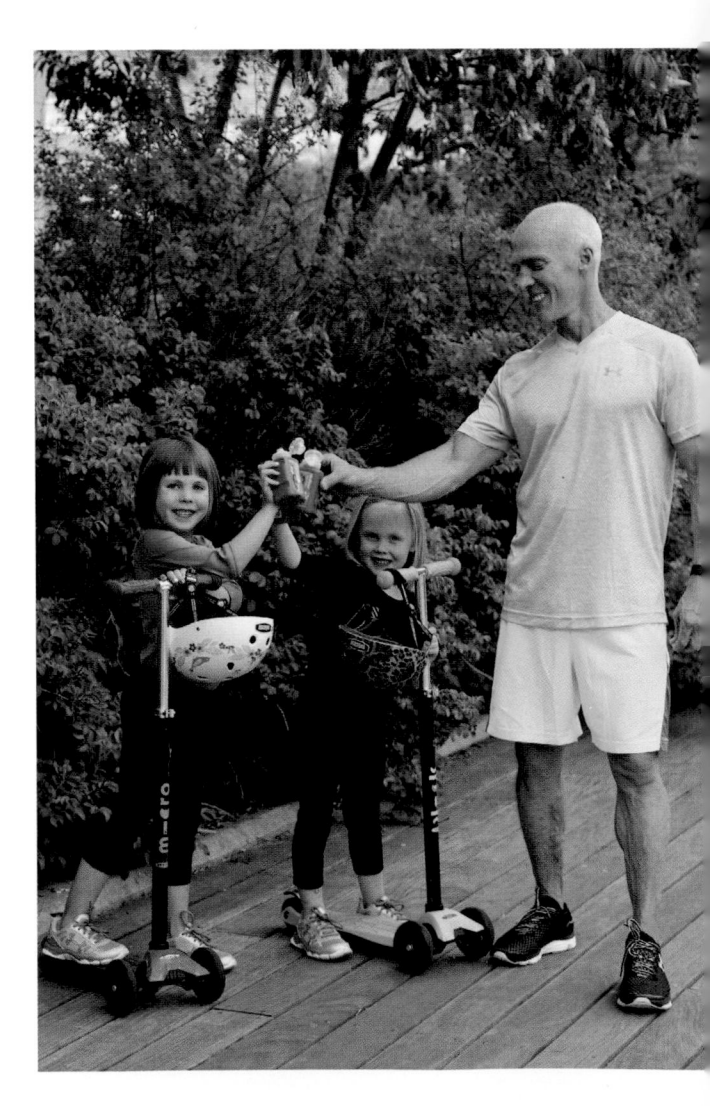

you realize your best you. The fitness portion of the program turns ordinary daily activities into mini fitness/wellness sessions: The family bicycle trip around the park, the pick-up soccer game, or the scooter ride to the grocery store—they are all invaluable moments of movement. So, whether you are doing a lower body routine of squats, lunges, and platypus walks or jumping jacks, shadow boxing, and pushups, your family can easily join in.

For me, the key to successfully juggling the roles of single father, fitness/wellness entrepreneur, and former exercise junky is prioritizing. Gone are the energizing, solitary sixty-minute workouts. Now I rely on five-minute workouts—and they're just as effective.

You may read this and say, "What can you truly accomplish in just five minutes a day, for five days?" The answer is simple—*a lot*! Research has shown that the type of high-intensity interval training you'll do as part of the 5-5-5 Program is a form of cardiovascular exercise. These short, intensive workouts will improve your athletic capacity and condition, glucose metabolism, and fat-burning potential.

I have also learned to adapt and create opportunities to include and expose Emilia and Francesca to exercise. As soon as they could walk (or at least balance on my back), I started organically sharing fitness moments with them, and now exercise is a natural, fun part of their lives.

You'll see in this book beautiful pictures of them squatting, lunging, and working up a sweat in the cardio room of the Madison Square Club gym, of Francesca adding weight to Liv Tyler's pushups, of Ellen Barkin squatting and holding four-month-old Emilia and Francesca, of Francesca not only challenging and beating Kate Upton in a pushup contest but also competing with Gigi Hadid on the rowing machine.

New Nutrition

We will also focus on your nutritional intake, which is of utmost importance. You will find delicious and nutritious five-ingredient recipes that take no more than fifteen minutes to prepare, including healthy recipes for breakfast, lunch, dinner, sides, snacks, smoothies, and juices. I've also revised and updated my well-established "ABCs of Nutrition" and expanded them to include F (fiber), G (dark leafy greens and whole grains), H (herbs), and S (seeds). Finally, I reveal the previously unheralded benefits of cooking with fresh herbs, offer up an extensive pantry list for stocking your healthy kitchen, and debunk some all-too-common food myths.

Once you've digested all the basics, you'll see that wellness builds exponentially. I have experienced firsthand the importance of raising healthy babies and have watched Emilia and Francesca grow into healthy toddlers and healthy beautiful six-year-old girls. Young girls, mind you, that are able to navigate grocery stores and farmers' markets better than many adults.

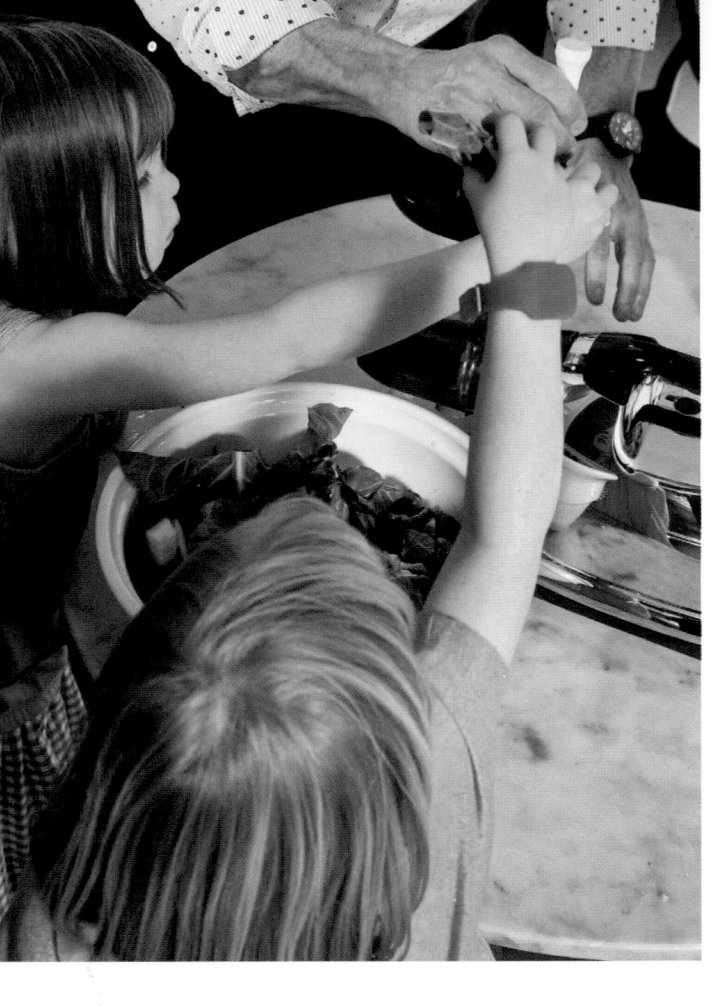

Of course, we enjoy our gelato as an occasional treat, too, but we also love roasting a head of cauliflower and drinking a healthy green juice and smoothie. We love cuddling on the sofa to a good movie (our favorite right now is *Charlotte's Web*), but you'll also find us "killing it" on the scooter to school, playing tennis, or going for a swim.

Management and Maintenance Made Easy

In the final chapter, you'll get five day-by-day trackers for the plan's meals and exercise. Plus, I'll show you how simple and easy it will be to maintain your impressive results. Unlike other fitness books out there, this program doesn't end at the completion of the five days. Once you've finished your exercises—sumoed, squatted, and planked to shape, tone, and sculpt your body— you'll be *armed* (see what I did there?) with the confidence and knowledge you need to adapt an everyday fitness program to your daily routine. You'll find suggested meal plans, online resources, and more.

The 5-5-5 Program is not a "one size fits all" program. Consistent with my overall philosophy, the program can be tailored to different body types and family needs. It allows for some necessary gelato splurges *and* gives you plenty of fun, organic moments to play with your children while keeping everyone in great shape.

Let's Get Cooking

My objective is to show you how easy these nutritional changes can be for you and your family. I make cooking fun (no, really!) because if it's not fun, it won't happen. I get it. My girls love to cook with me. Why? Because it's not a chore, it's an event. The girls have become pretty proficient in the kitchen, too. Francesca cracks a mean egg, and both girls like flipping their (gluten-free) French toast on the stove. Just this morning, the girls helped me make our breakfast—Oatmeal Banana Brulee (see page 153). We enjoyed it that much more knowing we all had a hand in preparing the delicious outcome.

NOW GET GOING!

Knowing what you can do in just five minutes a day for five days, are you ready to transform your life? Are you ready to transform your family's life? Whether completing one of the customized circuit workouts, preparing healthy meals with your children, or going on a family bike ride, The Ultimate Family Wellness Plan will improve the quality of your family's life immeasurably in the following ways:

- You will look and feel better. As advertised, you will lose up to five pounds using the program outlined in chapter 5, increasing your energy levels and improving your focus.

- You will have increased self-confidence and the tools to maintain and build upon your impressive initial results.

- You will learn to prepare fast and easy nutrient-rich meals.

- You will learn the principles for a sound mind and sound body to help you live a less-stressed, happier, and more productive life.

What are you waiting for? The time is now!

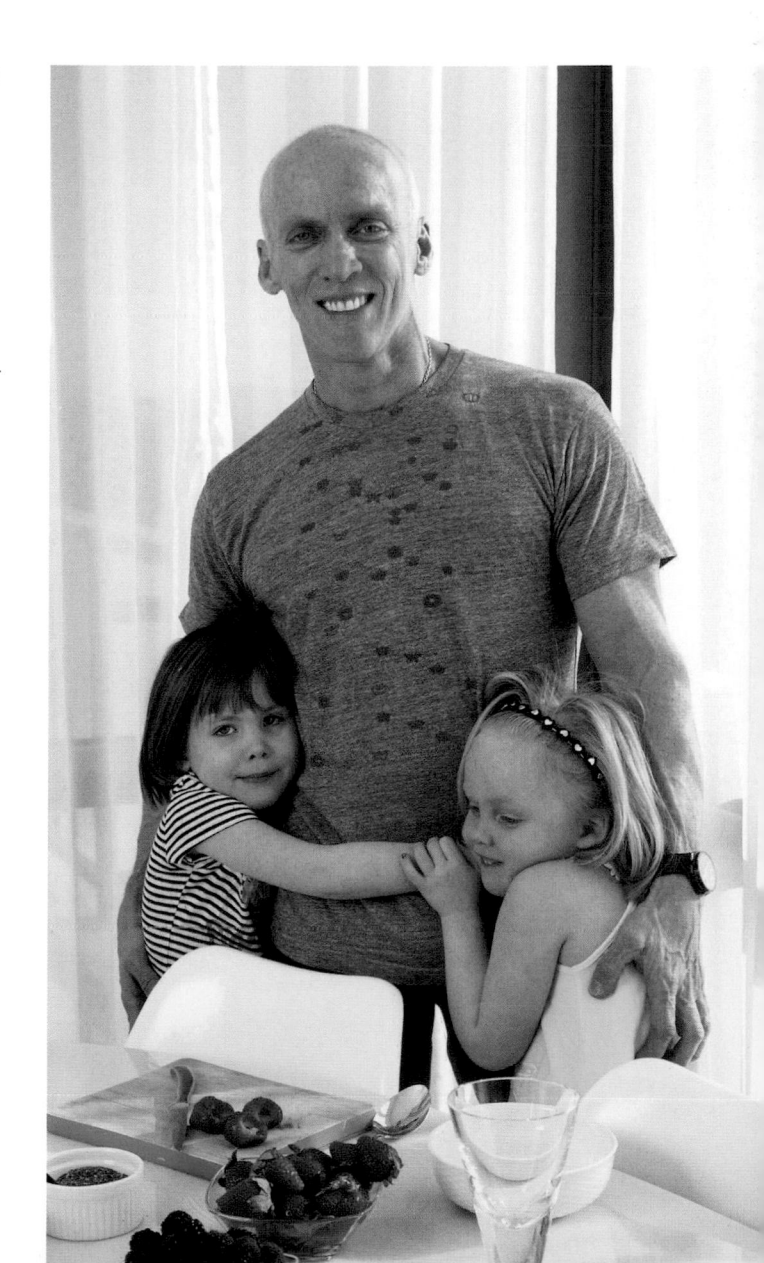

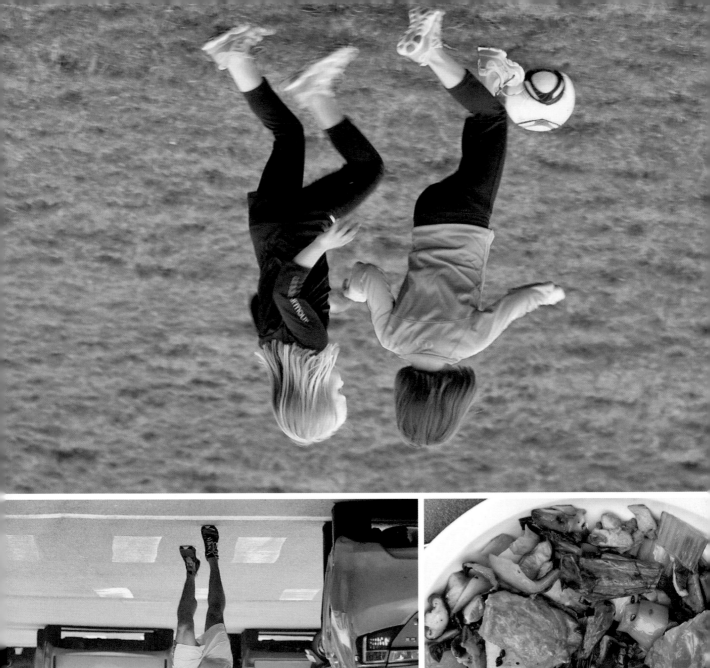
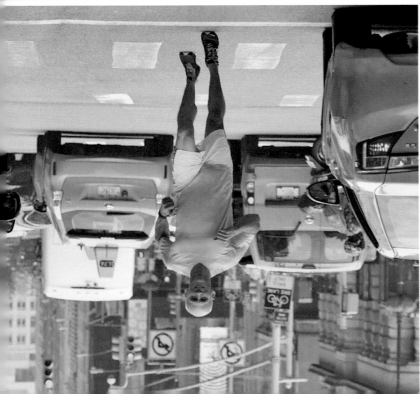
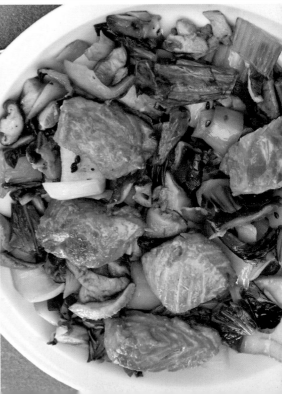

Chapter 1

WHAT IS THE 5-5-5 PROGRAM AND THE ULTIMATE FAMILY WELLNESS PLAN?

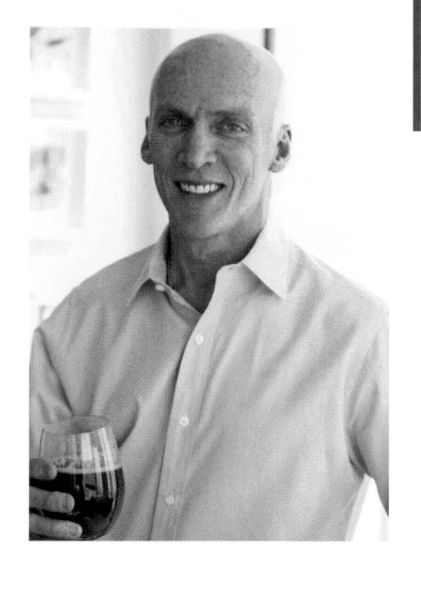

WELCOME TO THE 5-5-5 PROGRAM

David Kirsch's 5-5-5 Program didn't start as a family fitness and wellness program. Lose five pounds in five days? That was born out of a simple, yet challenging concept: five moves, five days, five pounds. Over the years, I've been known to "work magic" for any number of reasons—a magazine cover, a red carpet event, a movie scene or catwalk, or even a hot new date. Modeling agencies, movie studios, models, actors, and ordinary men and women keep me on speed dial for those special, time-crunched moments.

Using a combination of my signature exercises with compound movements and short bursts of cardiovascular exercise, all performed as a five-minute circuit (more specifics on this a little later in this chapter), you can rev up your metabolism, tone and shape muscles, and increase your overall energy. Add to that my A to H "Rules of Nutrition," and you have a recipe for the perfect start to a new you. The program, found in chapter 5, will increase your energy levels and give you greater mind-body awareness.

How does a five-day weight-loss and tune-up program weave into the daily fabric of everyday family life to become the Ultimate Family Wellness Plan? Its accessibility, affordability, adaptability, and overall ease of use allow it to transcend from personal health to the perfect family fitness and wellness plan.

Losing those first five pounds—especially in just five days—can motivate you to feel great and incorporate a new nutrition and fitness philosophy into your day-to-day life. During the program's five days, you'll reconnect with your body; learn a simple, delicious, diverse way to eat; and master

straightforward exercises you can do anytime, anywhere. You can always return to the program if you need to lose those "stubborn" five pounds in a hurry, but the real value is in the core concepts you will acquire and the effect on your family— that essential idea that wellness is universal and meant for everyone. It only takes a few minutes and a few movements to reshape your overall wellness and transform you and those around you.

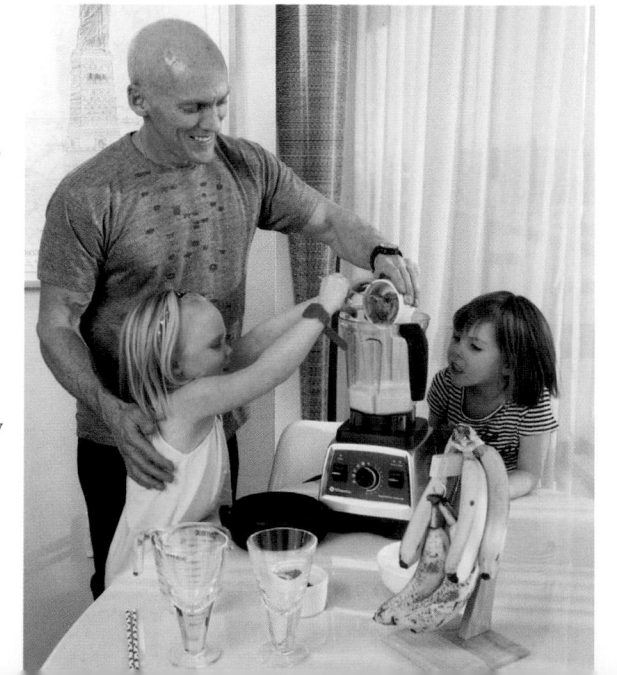

WHAT IS THE ULTIMATE FAMILY WELLNESS PLAN?

Lessons we learn as young children help form the foundation for the rest of our lives—our relationship with food, exercise, body awareness, body image, and self-confidence. The principles of healthy eating, snacking, and daily exercise are ageless and invaluable. With the suggestions in this book for easily achievable adjustments to your outlook on eating—which includes delicious, easy-to-follow (not to mention kid-friendly) recipes such as almond pancakes and my tasty and fun egg-and-spinach muffins—and family-friendly physical activities such as cycling or scooter rides, any family can become the Ultimate Fit Family.

As you're starting to see, the 5-5-5 Program leads to so much more than weight loss; it is a lifestyle philosophy that will forever transform how you and your family view diet and exercise. This became abundantly clear when I shot the photographs for this book with my daughters Emilia and Francesca. When I asked them whether they wanted photos of us cooking and exercising together included in the book, they responded with a resounding, "Yes!" The first shoot took place on Super Bowl weekend, in my two favorite places: my apartment kitchen and my gym, the Madison Square Club. I watched with great pride (and truth be told, amazement) as both girls exceeded all expectations.

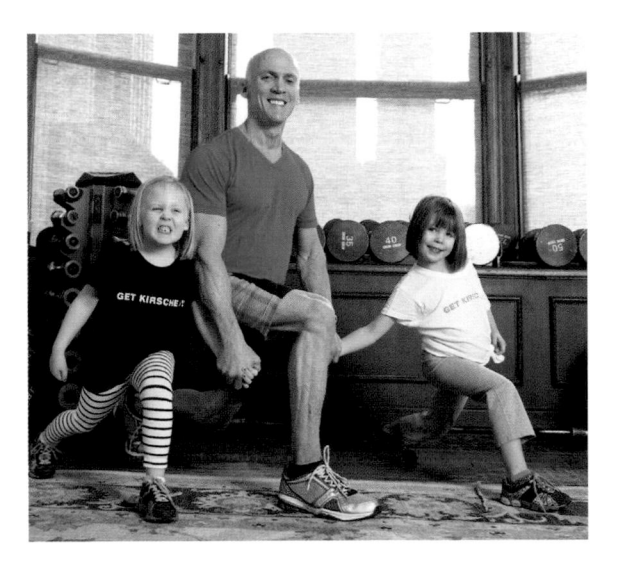

It is one thing to write about family wellness and quite another to see it unfold so organically before my eyes. Here were my beautiful five-and-a-half-year-old daughters sharing my passion for healthy living—helping me prepare quick and tasty banana chocolate peanut butter smoothies, yogurt parfaits, and Oatmeal Banana Brulee. The next day we shot the exercise pictures. As you can see from the amazing photos, Emilia and Francesca enjoyed sharing their favorite exercises. After two days and twenty hours of shooting, they were still laughing and enjoying every moment. I was proud of them, and most importantly, they were proud of themselves. This is what my Ultimate Family Wellness Plan is all about.

GETTING STARTED ON THE 5-5-5 PROGRAM

Now that you know the Ultimate Family Wellness Plan is not a diet but rather a way of life, where do you start? Below is an overview of what you can expect from the 5-5-5 Program (work for five days, lose five pounds), found in chapter 5, and how you can turn that supercharged start into a fitter, healthier lifestyle. Before we get there, let's get in the right mindset.

The Time is Now

When I was researching this chapter, I remembered a piece I wrote for *The Huffington Post* in July 2014, titled, "The Time is Now." It seems a simple-enough phrase, but all too often, I hear people living in the past or future. So much of our lives is uncertain. We're born with the power to manifest greatness, yet somewhere along the way, we get sidetracked. Why do some people succeed while for others, success futilely slips by? As a fitness and wellness expert for more than a quarter century, I have helped many men and women realize their wellness goals. That's not to say I haven't had my share of clients who, try as I might and sweat as they should, failed to realize or maintain their wellness goals. The difference between success and failure is often so slight, yet seemingly so unattainable.

Before you embark on a fitness and wellness regime, you need a plan of action. You need the following four steps:

1 A set of realistic goals

2 A timeline

3 A fitness and nutrition program that suits your lifestyle

4 Motivation and behavior modification

The first three points are quite obvious, on the surface, and easy to identify. The final bullet, motivation and behavior modification, is often difficult to harness and overcome. Failure to recognize and implement all four steps will sabotage even the surest wellness plan. There's a kind of symbiosis between motivation and behavior—when both are in sync, they make "beautiful music." However, behavioral aspects of your personality are often mired in the past—self-doubt, self-loathing, and self-worth: "I can't work out." "It's too difficult to eat healthy food." "I'll never look like _____." Turn the negative into positive affirmations: "I will try my best to move my body every day." "I will be mindful of what I eat and drink." "I will strive to love my best self."

Many people live their lives like robots, going through the motions at work and in their relationships. They feel little inner passion. It's not that the passion isn't there; they simply do not tap into it. If only they could unleash their passion, their lives would become more fulfilling.

People often fear passion. It is misunderstood and sometimes applied in the wrong way. But the clearer your path and the stronger your passion, the greater your chances of success. Inner passion clarifies life, makes it easier and meaningful. When you live with passion, everything falls into place, freeing energy for you to pursue your wellness goals of eating healthily and exercising. We all have to find our passion, strive for the best, and most importantly, live a fulfilled life that exudes goodness and spirituality. We are all born with amazing possibilities and potential.

I have suffered much adversity in my life. Once I realized the precious nature of time, I decided my life was too short to waste on negativity. True, every so often I have a bad day and feel down because of it. But rarely do I allow myself to stay down for long. It's a waste of time, and I'm in better health because of it. I am also blessed with the two most amazing daughters—my little angels—and just a smile and hug from Emilia and Francesca is enough to lift me out of the darkest place.

Negative emotions—anger, jealousy, depression, frustration, worry, anxiety, you name it—drain your energy and put you at a higher risk for disease. Some things are worth feeling sad about, but many are not. Find a way to get your inner peace in order.

How do you change your emotions? You do it by slowing down, noticing them, and taking corrective action. The Chinese have a phrase, *pu shih*, which means you accept what comes in life, whether you perceive it as positive or negative. You create negative emotions when you fight this acceptance. Once you embrace this philosophy, as I have, you will see that anything is possible. When you meet a barrier—any barrier—examine it, break it down into steps, and deal with it one step at a time.

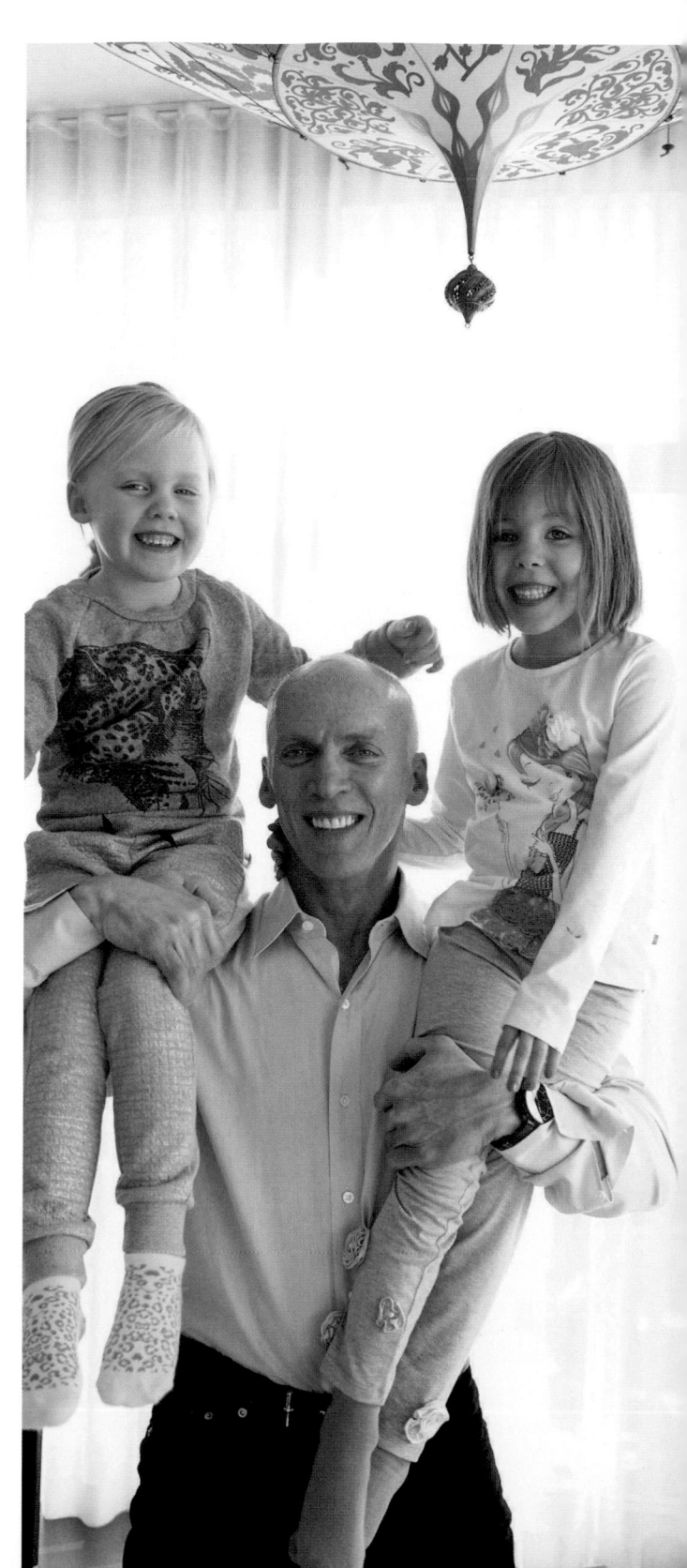

FIVE DAYS TO LOSE FIVE POUNDS—AND BEYOND

Now that you know the benefits of the 5-5-5 Program and understand the importance of motivation, let's talk about what you can expect. During the plan's five days, you won't count calories, weigh portions, or anything like that. You will eat healthful whole foods, including proteins and greens.

The Five Rules for Optimal Nutrition on page 116 will lay it all out for you, and the recipe chapter, chapter 4, will offer every dish you will make on those five days. They're so delicious and nourishing, I am confident you'll cook them for a long time after that as well.

You will also do five minutes of HIIT (high-intensity interval training—more on that below) every day to reconnect body and mind and recalibrate your body. These exercises will burn fat, build strength, sculpt muscles, and boost metabolism. I'm a firm believer, however, that there is no universal exercise plan. Different body types need different programs to get the best results. That's why I've tailored the workouts (see chapter 2) to three different body types:

- weight carried in the lower body (i.e., hips, thighs, and glutes)

- weight carried in the upper body (i.e., back, belly, and arms)

- weight carried evenly all over

These exercises are so fast and effective, that, like the recipes, I believe you'll use them for a long time after the initial five days. They are largely body-weight exercises and therefore require no special equipment. A medicine ball or kettle bell, stability ball, and some light weights are all you need, and you can usually find suitable substitutes at home for items you don't have.

For the day-by-day meal and exercise plans, see page 202 in chapter 5.

Why HIIT?

High-intensity interval training (HIIT) is a technique that requires you to give everything you've got for short, intense bursts of exercise, followed by periods of rest. Research has shown that this method, which pushes you practically to your limit for a short time, is more effective than doing long sessions of cardio. The intensity (and it is intense!) boosts your metabolism by using up more oxygen than your body can take in. Your body then keeps consuming higher levels of oxygen to make up for the deficit, burning fat well after the workout ends.

Studies even show that HIIT can help improve cardiovascular health, increase stamina, and control glucose levels. Though people once thought HIIT was only okay for athletes, more research keeps coming out showing myriad health benefits for people with chronic health problems such as diabetes, pulmonary disease, arthritis, and for those recovering from strokes. Plus, it's excuse-proof, requiring little time and no specialized equipment.

WELLNESS ROLE MODEL

With new health-and-fitness knowledge in hand, your family will learn simply by watching you eat well and exercise. As you make it a part of your life, it will naturally become a part of their lives, too, giving them invaluable lessons about health, well-being, and body image they will carry with them forever. Wellness is the ultimate gift you can give to yourself and your loved ones, and with this program, you can share that gift by bonding over delicious and nourishing food, fun exercises, and a happy, healthy attitude that connects mind and body.

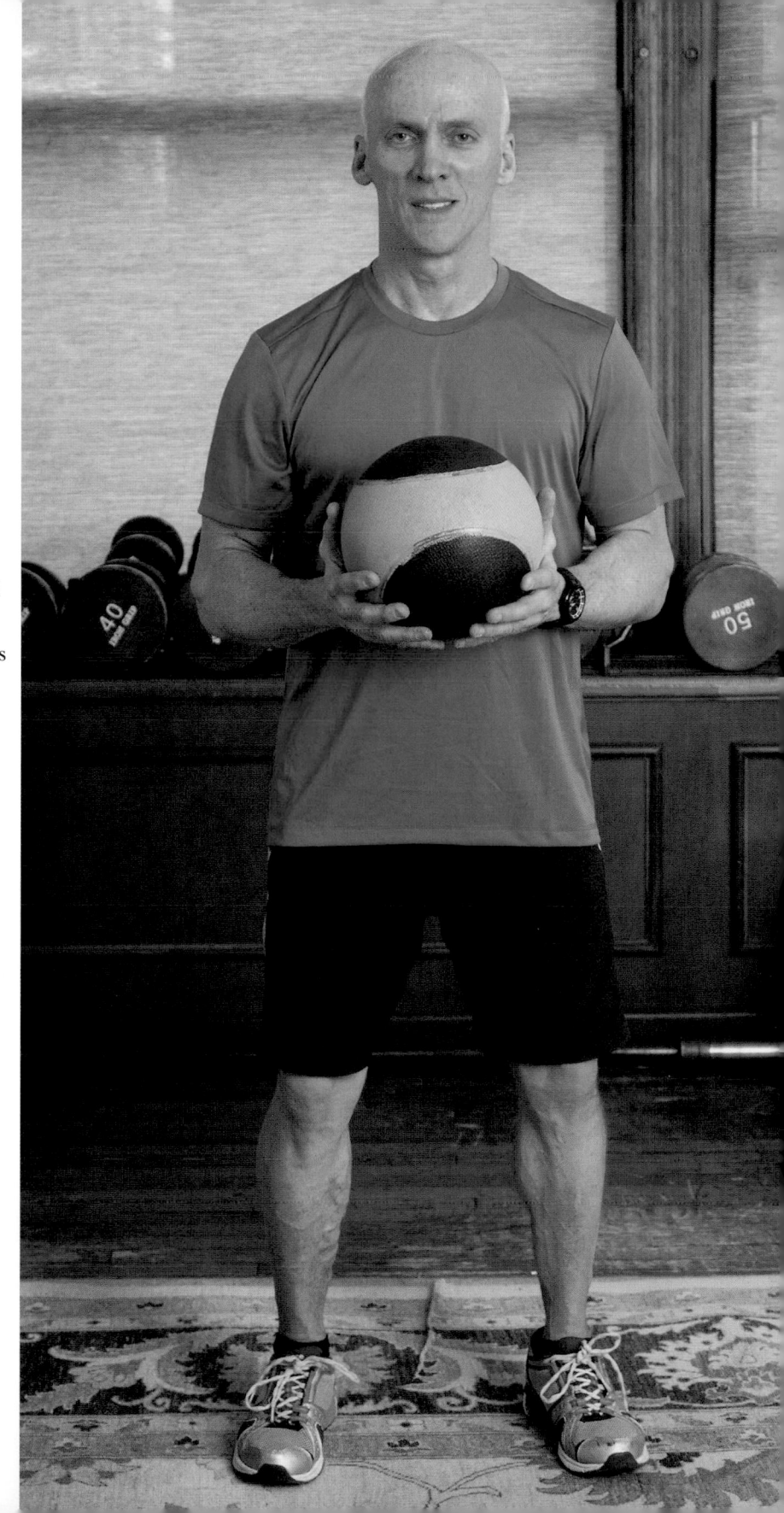

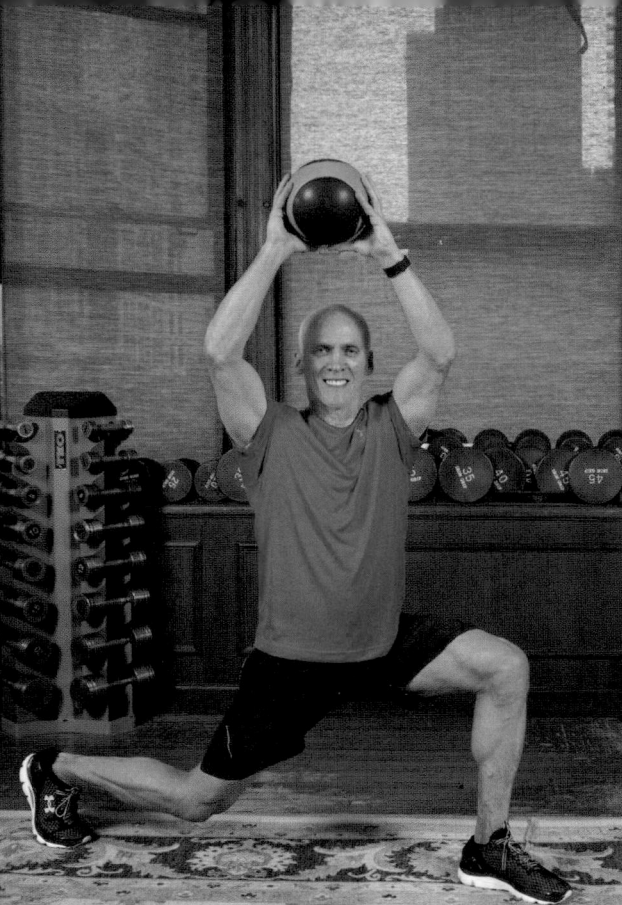
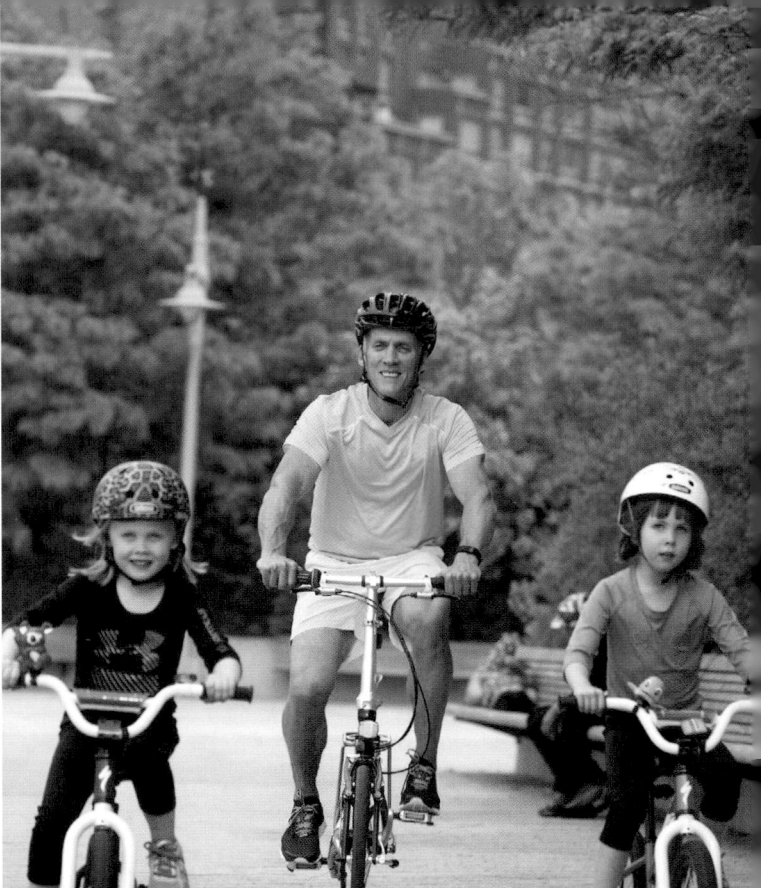

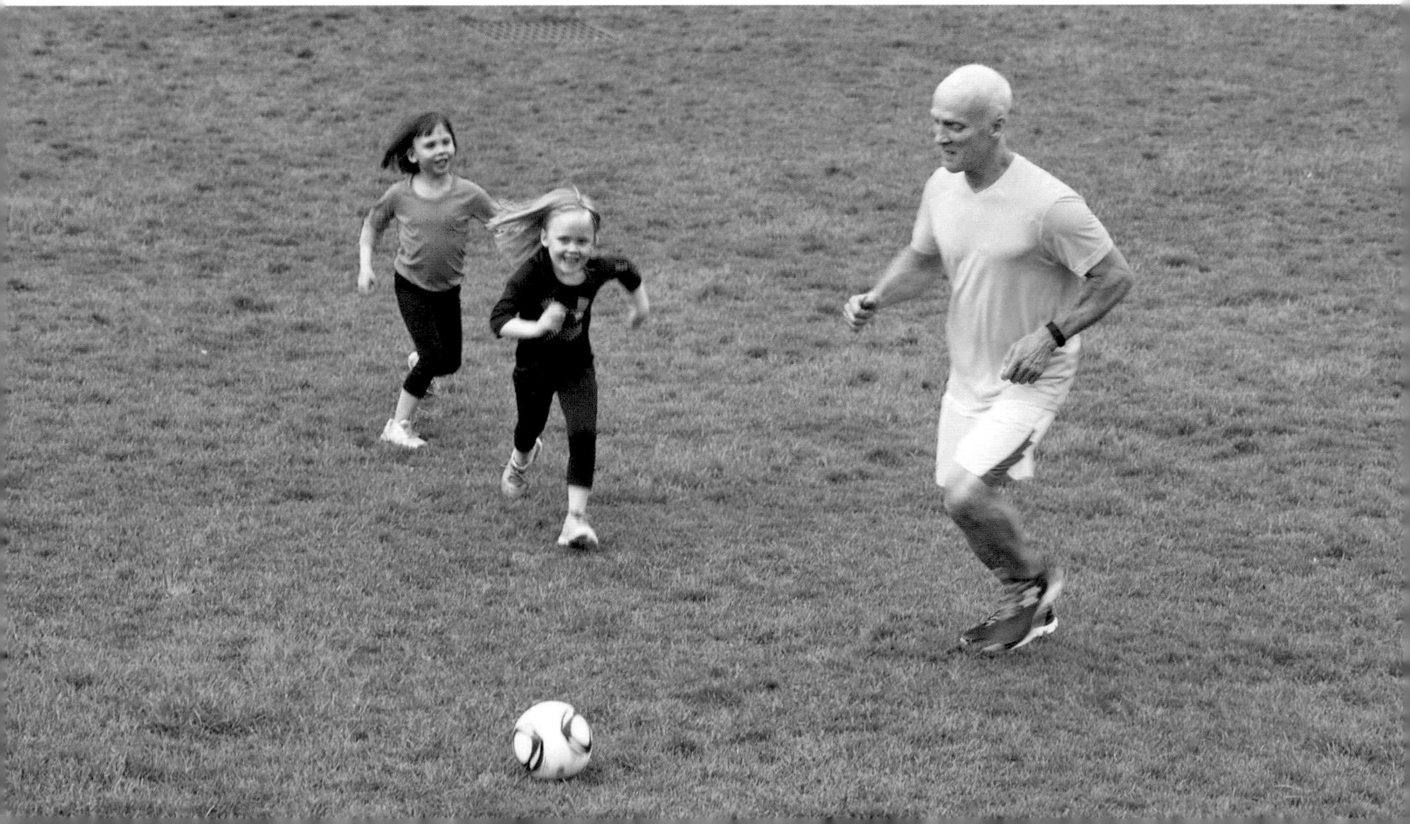

Chapter 2

EXERCISING AND ACTIVITIES

EXERCISES FOR THE 5-5-5 PROGRAM

I have always believed that there isn't a "one size fits all" exercise prescription. I generally break down the body into three distinct groups:

1 The person who carries weight in his or her hips, thighs, and butt

2 The person who carries weight in her or her back, arms, and belly

3 The person with evenly distributed weight

Your body type will determine which five-exercise David Kirsch Express Workout you should perform for the five-day, five-pound weight-loss plan (see chapter 5) and in your new Ultimate Family Wellness lifestyle. (I will also give you a total-body plank workout that anyone can do regardless of location or time constraints.) Remember, these exercises are not just for five days of weight loss; they're exercises you can do anywhere, any time, to keep up your strength and energy.

Not only is this program fully customizable, offering you specific exercises that will help you target "trouble spots" (pet peeves), it is also excuse-proof, as it can be done anywhere, any time, with no more than body-weight resistance (no special equipment required).

Is the family at home? No worries. Many exercises in this book are family-friendly. As you will see throughout this book, Emilia, Francesca, and I often exercise together. We feel great when we do it, and it's a great way to share my passion for fitness, spend time together, and bond.

Later, we will explore a whole range of activities that your children won't even realize are exercise. Exercise is movement and movement is fun. When exercising with your kids, always use your best judgment about what your child can and cannot do. I will let you know when an exercise is child-friendly but overall, children can try most of the movements in this book. If they're still young, they'll have fun simply trying. Emilia and Francesca often come to the gym to help me train my clients. Teenagers will likely be able to do the exercises every bit as well as you can (if not better). But never push your children too hard and never forget, the most important part to getting them hooked on fitness is making it fun.

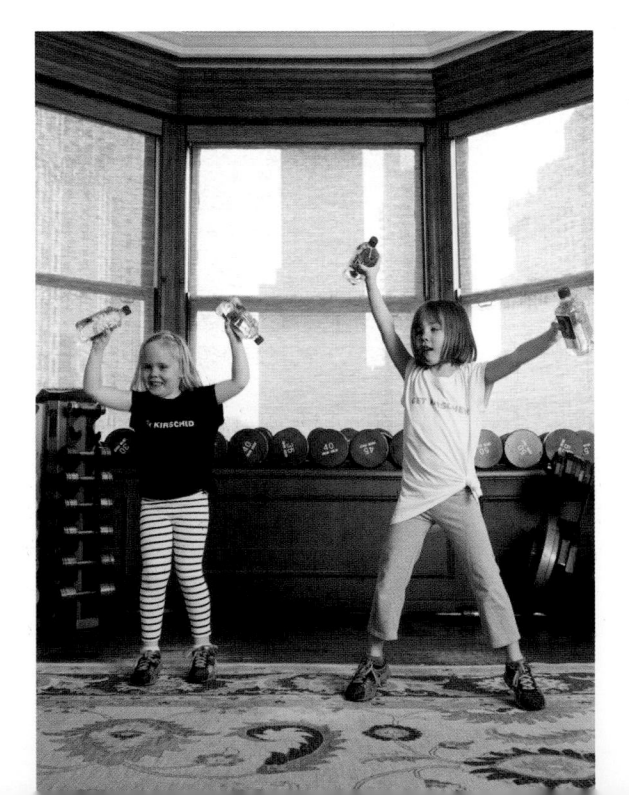

MAKING WORKOUTS FAILPROOF

Before we get into the exercises themselves, I want to address a few questions and concerns I get all the time. I've spent the better part of a quarter century (more than half my life) dedicated to health, fitness, and wellness. In that time, the most frequently asked question would have to be: Why isn't my workout plan working? If you're reading this book, there's a chance that what you've been doing is not getting the hoped-for results, and you're ready for something different. If you're new to fitness, this will ensure that you start on the right foot and get the most out of your workouts.

There isn't one simple answer to why a workout plan fails or plateaus before real results show. The following suggestions are those I have shared with clients, followers, friends, and family alike, to great success.

You don't have a proper plan.

Workouts often start and fail in the planning (or lack thereof) stage. Before you take your first step, ask yourself the "what, why, and for whom" of your routine. What do you hope to accomplish? Why are you doing this and for whom? Simply put, for a diet and exercise program to be successful, you need a specific goal (e.g., lose weight, tone up) and a clear course of action (i.e., the right program) to fit your lifestyle and budget.

Last but not least, make sure you are doing this for yourself and not someone else. Doing it for someone else will leave you feeling resentful and unfulfilled and ultimately sabotage and undermine the possibility of realizing your wellness goals. Once you've satisfactorily answered the "what, why, and for whom," set a realistic goal and timeline.

You aren't in the moment.

In my book *Sound Mind, Sound Body*, I advise readers to take time out of their days to "honor" themselves. Here, I make that same recommendation. This is the time of day you dedicate to your wellness. Make every moment of those five-minute exercise circuits count. When you physically leave the office, mentally leave the office behind. Turn off your cell phone. (Full disclosure: I take my phone onto the workout floor. As a single father, I need to be connected at all times of the day. However, save the crazy emergency, I try to avoid looking at it. As I am always running against the clock, my workout time is precious to me.)

Workout time is not time to socialize, catch up on your soap operas, or Google Chat with your friends. Too often I see people "walking through" their workouts, which can lead to injury, unrealized goals, and ultimately complete dissatisfaction with a training routine. To make the most out of your workouts, stay focused, engage your brain, and visualize the body you were meant to have. Want it, will it, and make it happen.

You don't get enough sleep.

Failure to get adequate sleep will, among other things, leave you feeling depleted mentally and physically and will sabotage your hard-earned workout gains. It can elevate your cortisol levels, which can lead to weight gain. Lastly, poor eating habits and sleep deprivation usually go hand in hand. When you feel tired, you often make bad food choices (e.g., eat comfort foods because they're convenient rather than healthy foods).

You don't get proper fuel.

I like to say "Eat to live." Starving your body will only serve to upend your fitness/wellness transformation. You need a balanced diet. Fill up on fruits, vegetables, grains, lean proteins, legumes, nuts, and seeds. Small, abundant healthful meals throughout the day will keep you optimally fueled and keep your brain, organs, and body working efficiently.

Good Form Means Great Results

I have always been known as a stickler for the physiology and mechanics of every exercise. To maximize your workout results, you need to know how your body should look and feel with proper exercise form, and conversely, how it shouldn't look and feel.

There are many different types of exercises for every part of your body. That said, the execution of these exercises plays an integral role in your overall success. When training clients, I often catch myself saying, both as a question and a directive, "Feel the difference." I use this as a tool to correct the mechanics of an exercise and to remind clients to connect mind and body during exercise. In the following paragraphs, I will illustrate this philosophy for each major muscle group.

Visualization, or the art of seeing what you are trying to accomplish, will help you maintain the mind-body connection throughout each exercise. Your ability to visualize will in part determine the effectiveness of your workout. See it, feel it, and make it happen.

The core is a great example. Sit up straight. We've all heard this from our parents, teachers, and adults in our lives. Now I find myself saying this to my daughters, clients, and anyone I catch slouching. To me, the core is the most important part of your body and one that is often and easily neglected. Engage your core! What does this mean? The core is so much more than just the belly.

It begins with proper postural alignment. Sit (or stand) up tall, shoulders back and shoulder blades retracted (i.e., back and pulled together). Pull your belly button in towards your spine.

Failure to engage your core can compromise an exercise, put unnecessary strain on your lower back, and at the extreme, cause musculoskeletal damage. I do believe in the adage that "abs are made in the kitchen," but I would add they're punctuated during your workout. Keeping your core engaged offers innumerable benefits and doing so will serve you well for years to come. Whether you are sitting at your desk, power walking, doing abdominal work, or even doing lunges and squats, you need to maintain postural integrity and engage your core.

Here are some tips for connecting your mind with other parts of your body and using the correct form for basic movements (they make up much of the customized exercises later in this chapter):

1. Sit-ups/Crunches. Feeling it in your neck? Cradle your head in your arms and keep your eyes focused straight above you. Feeling it in your lower back? Engage your core. Press your lower back into the mat (or floor) and visualize pulling your belly button in toward your spine. If you have musculoskeletal issues, try performing partial range-of-motion (ROM) crunches.

These days, I actually prefer plank exercises to strengthen and tone my core and abs. As you will see later in the book, I created an intense, effective circuit of five plank exercises that not only focus on strengthening and toning your core, but the rest of your body as well. Kate Upton, among others, is a huge fan of this circuit workout and uses it when she's on the road.

2. Pushups. Are you feeling it in your lower back? You're dropping your hips and not engaging your core. Are you feeling it in your neck and/or shoulders? You are engaging your traps (the trapezius muscles, which connect your neck to your shoulders and spine) and shoulders by lifting your shoulders up toward your ears. Those are the wrong muscles. The perfect push-up uses your chest, triceps, and core.

To perform the perfect pushup, start in the up position of a plank with your core engaged. Lift your shoulders and drop them back and down, retracting (i.e., pinching together) your shoulder blades. Place your hands about shoulder-width apart and directly under your chest. As you descend toward the ground, keep your shoulders down and drive the energy from your hands to your chest and triceps. Beginners can do partial ROM push-ups on your knees or against a wall, desk, or bench. This builds up your strength, stamina, and confidence. In no time, you will be doing regular pushups. One of the better teaching moments I've seen as a trainer happened when I was training Kate Upton. Emilia and Francesca were keeping us company and counting repetitions. Kate was doing pushups, but not really giving it her all, when Francesca said, "I can do that, daddy!" Francesca schooled Kate in how to do ten perfect pushups on her hands and toes.

3. Squats. Are you feeling it in your lower back? Engage your core, affix your eyes slightly upward, and do not arch your back. Are you feeling it in your knees? Your knees are extending past your toes. To ensure a proper and effective squat, Put Your Brain in Your Butt®. Anchor in your heels and drive the energy through your heels into your butt. To be safe, never go lower than your thighs parallel to the floor. Additionally, opt for dumbbell squats instead of barbell squats to avoid unnecessary strain on your lower back. They are a much safer, equally effective alternative.

4. Lunges. Are you feeling it in your knees? Your knees are extended past your toes. Use a mirror to correct your form until you get the hang of it. I want your legs to form two right angles in the completed stationery lunge. Are you feeling it in your quads alone and not your glutes? You're stepping onto the ball of your foot and not anchoring with your forward heel. When I lunge, I step into my heel and lean my torso slightly forward. Lunges (e.g., reverse, crossover, and lateral) help tone and sculpt your legs and butt-quads, hamstrings, and adductors (i.e., inner thighs). If you have issues with your knees, do partial ROM.

5. Shoulders. Are you feeling it in your traps and/or neck? Chances are you're engaging your traps (i.e., lifting and/or rotating forward) while you do shoulder presses and lateral or front raises. Before you begin, lift your shoulders and rotate back, retracting your shoulder blades. This will correct postural alignment and take the emphasis (and stress) out of your traps and neck.

6. Trapezius. I would advise against training your trapezius muscles, unless you are competitively bodybuilding or strength training. Given that point, you shouldn't engage or feel any exercises in your trapezius muscles. More than any other correction I make in the gym, I constantly remind my clients to relax their face and jaw and to disengage their traps—they are all related. Core engaging and scapulae retraction (i.e., shoulder blades pulled back and together) are what I remind my clients for proper pre-exercise alignment.

Now that you know the basics on form and the importance of connecting mind and body, let's get to your tailor-made David Kirsch Express Workout®. I will go into much more detail and provide illustrations and/or photographs of the correct form for each exercise, with tips on what not to do.

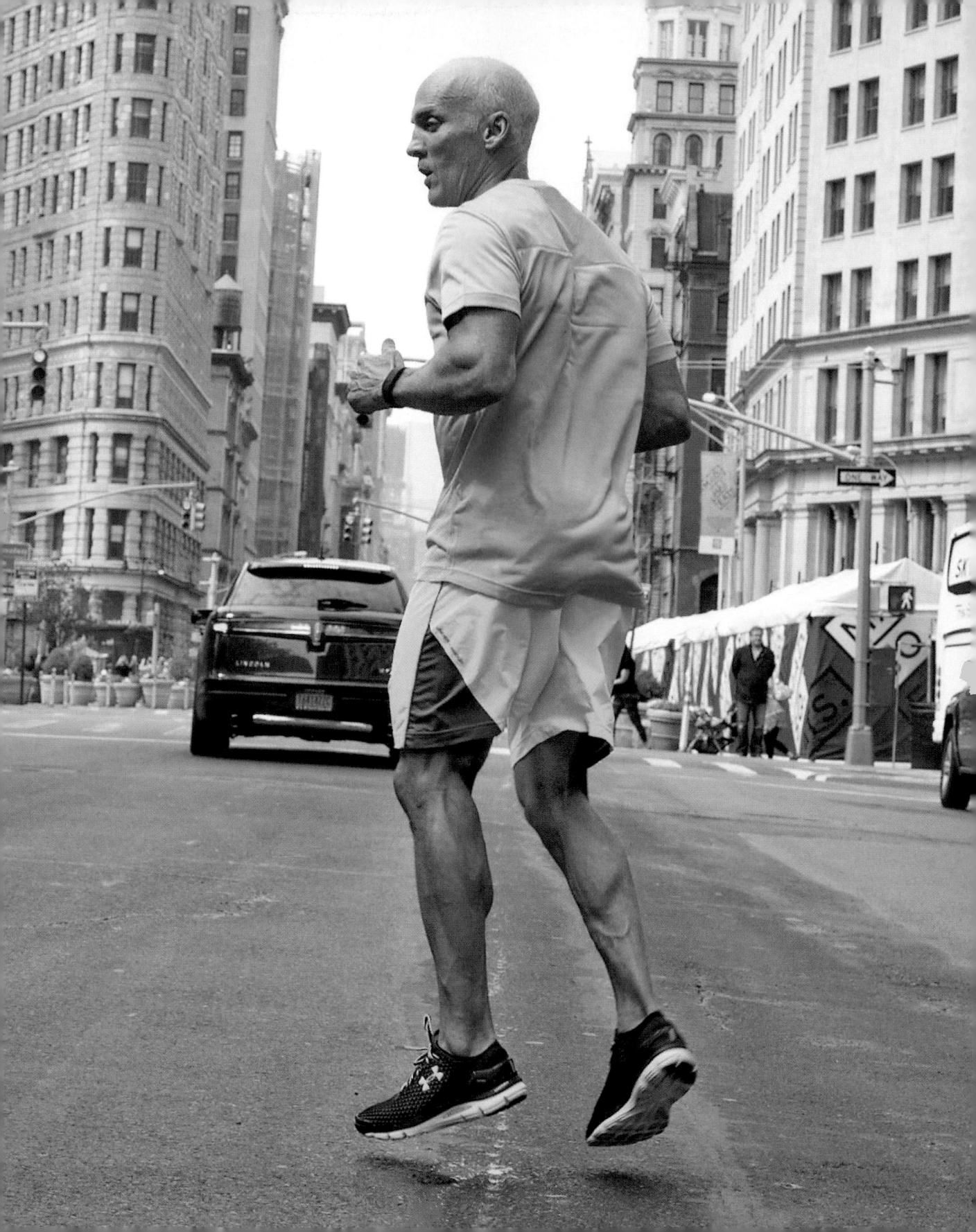

5-5-5 EXERCISES AND CUSTOMIZATION

Creating body-weight resistance exercises was one of the ways I made this program excuse-proof (we don't always have access or feel comfortable going to a gym). My training philosophy has always been to help you find your best you. As with all of my programs, this is meant as a guide. You'll use a specific menu of moves while on the five-day plan to lose five pounds (see chapter 5), but otherwise, feel free to personalize it to suit your physical condition and level of exercise. Over the years, I have found, used, and created signature exercises with just body-weight resistance, light to medium hand weights, or medicine balls. In my experience, you don't need heavy weights or machines to tone and sculpt your body, but rather just the exercises below, using the following method:

The five exercises will be performed as circuits. Each circuit is fifteen repetitions per side, without respite. You will repeat the circuit again, for a total of two circuits, with a thirty-second rest in between each circuit. This will total five minutes of exercise. As you build your strength and stamina, you may try to add a third set, making sure not to sacrifice form.

The adaptability of this program gives you license to repeat any of these five exercise circuits more than once daily. I find it particularly helpful and effective to sprinkle these circuits throughout my day. You could try a circuit in the middle of the day to get your body revving and your creative and productive juices flowing or at the end of the day as a way to de-stress and unwind. Let the following exercises of the 5-5-5 Program guide, inspire, and help direct you on your daily wellness plan. In fact, I just completed one of the full-body workouts, and let me tell you, it really works.

Finally, you will see that although this program is not designed for children, Emilia and Francesca are photographed throughout the book exercising, guiding, counting repetitions, and just having a good time. The key to the success of The Ultimate Family Wellness Plan and the 5-5-5 Program lies in its inclusiveness. Wellness begins at birth and grows and develops from there. Creating the Ultimate Wellness Family is the goal here, and this plan does just that; you will have fun in the most loving and bonding way. Wellness is now and forever—it has become an integral part of the fabric of my, Emilia's, and Francesca's life. Please join us on our journey—it will be life transformational.

LOWER BODY (Hips, Thighs, and Glutes)

For those who carry their weight in their legs, hips, thighs, and butt, the exercises in the 5-5-5 Program will concentrate on tightening, toning, lifting, and sculpting toner, sleeker thighs and a "perkier" butt. They don't call me the Master of the Ass® for nothing.

Now, I've said it before, but it is worth repeating: For optimal results when doing exercises for your lower body, put your brain in your butt®. To shape a better butt, place the focus and energy there and not in your quadriceps, lower back, or knees. I've put together a combination of plyometric and single-leg movements that will not only strengthen, tone, and sculpt your legs, but also work on your core balance and strength.

Sumo Lunge to a Side Kick with a Squat Jump

This is probably one of my most well known (and challenging) exercises. Perfected by Heidi Klum and me on the beach in the Hamptons, it is martial arts plus plyometrics and it equals a total thigh, hips, and butt blast. Here's how it works:

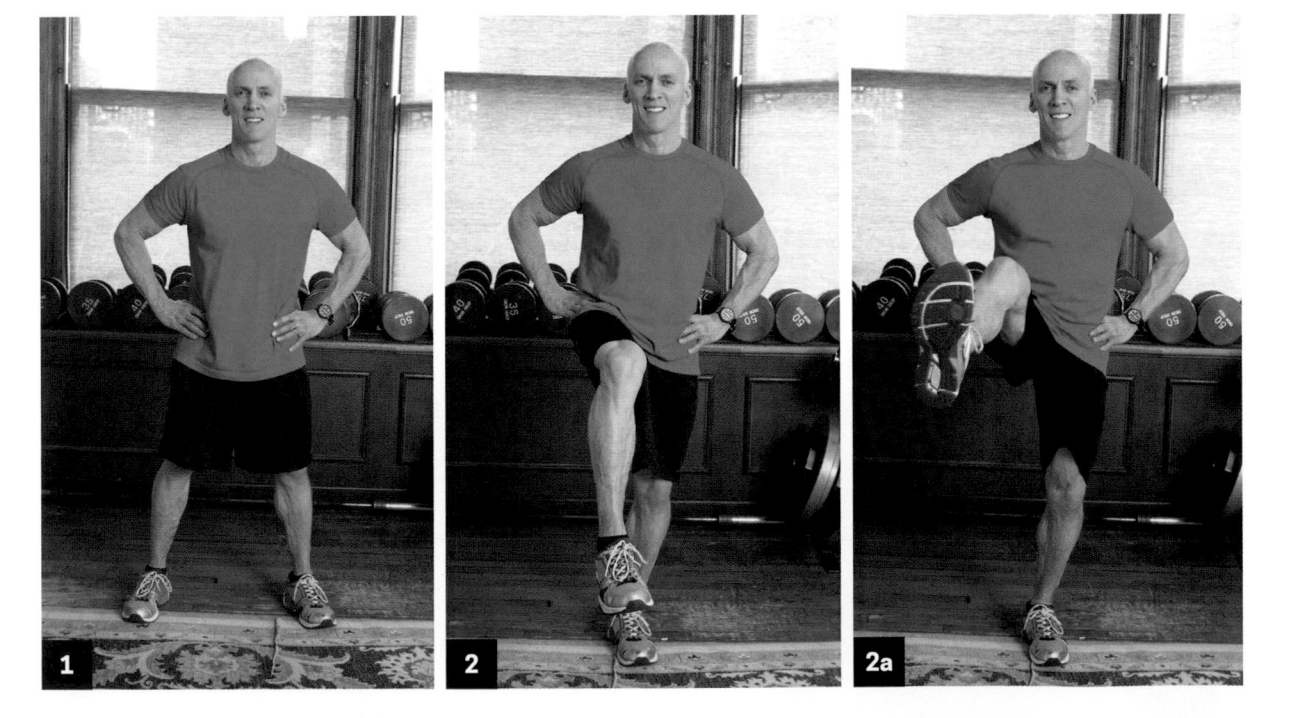

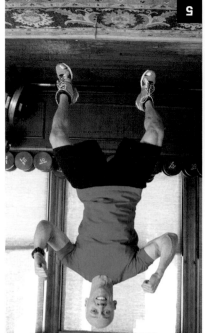

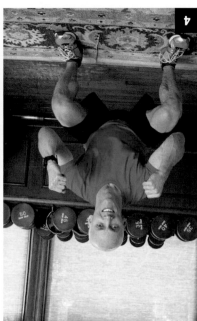

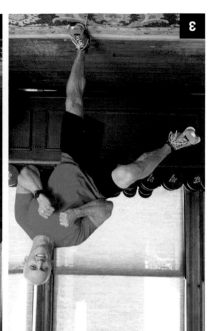

1 Stand in a "sumo" position with your feet slightly wider than shoulder-width apart, knees bent, and body weight over your heels.

2 Take a large step sideways with your right leg, bringing your right knee in toward your chest and then over to the right (2a) in one continuous movement.

3 As soon as your right foot touches the ground, bring your knee back into your chest and complete a side kick, kicking your right heel out to the side.

4 Lower your right leg to the floor, returning to sumo position. Squat down while keeping the weight in your heels and stick out your butt. Keep your knees directly above—not in front of—your toes.

5 Spring up while thrusting your arms overhead. Land on your heels, rolling forward onto your toes. Repeat with a sumo lunge and side kick with your left leg and another squat jump. Continue alternating right and left until you have completed fifteen lunges on each side and thirty squat jumps.

Single Leg Deadlifts

Tone and sculpt your inner thighs while shaping your butt with this balance-challenging exercise.

1 Start with your feet shoulder-width apart. Balancing on your right leg, bend at the waist and reach your left hand down to your right foot (1a); extend your left leg straight behind you (1b).

2 Keep both hips square (i.e., facing down) during the movement. Return to the starting position. That's one rep. Perform fifteen repetitions on each leg.

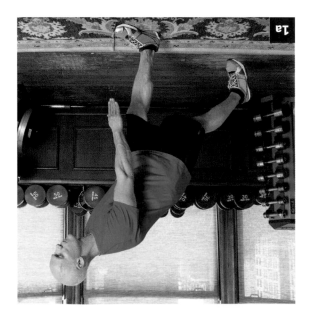

Plié Toe Squats

Take a wide stance, squat, and simultaneously raise up your heels so that you balance on your toes as you squat down. This will blast your inner thighs, butt, and core.

1 Start with your feet wider than shoulder-width apart and turned out at forty-five-degree angles with your hands on your hips. As you squat down, simultaneously lift up your heels as high as you can.

2 Return to starting position. That's one rep. Perform fifteen repetitions. This move is great for the otherwise hard-to-engage upper inner thigh (often referred to in magazines as thigh gap).

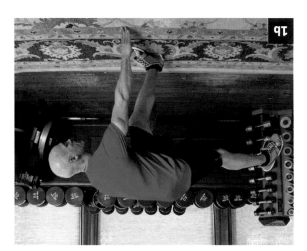

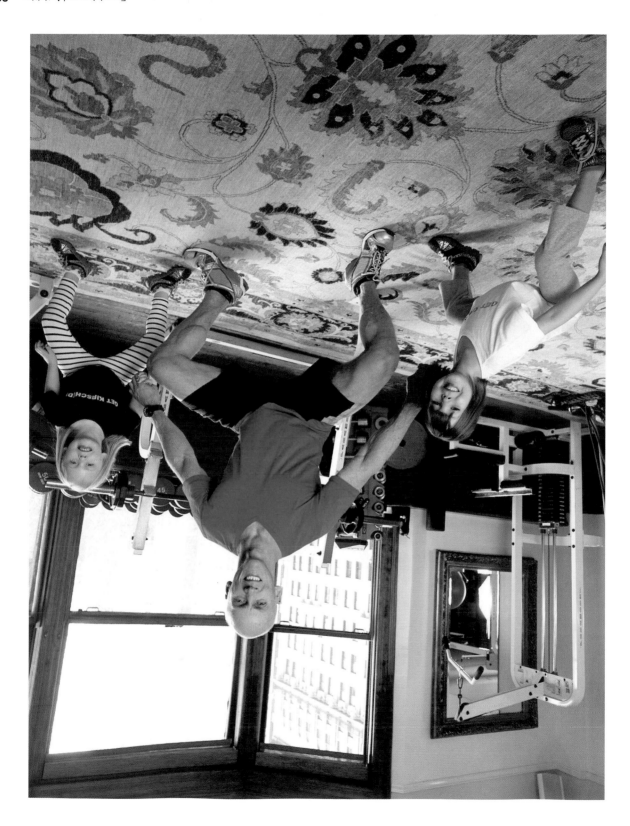

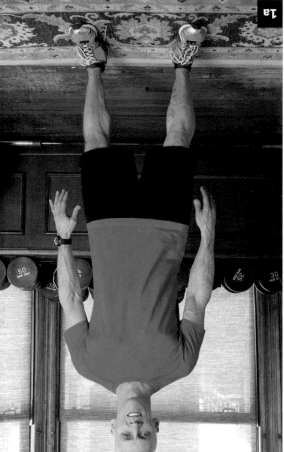

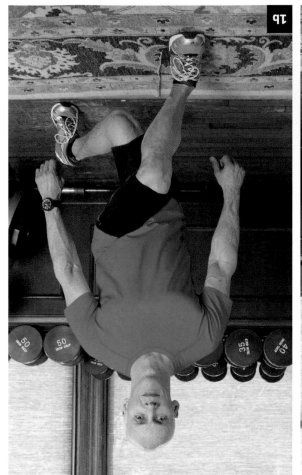

Reverse Crossover Lunge to Lateral Lunge

This great combination move will engage your inner and outer thighs, butt, and hips.

1 Stand with your feet shoulder-width apart (1a). Step your right leg back and behind your left leg and lunge, almost as if curtsying (1b).

2 Reverse to return to the starting position.

3 Step your right leg out to the side laterally, without pausing. Step into your right heel, keeping the right knee aligned with the heel. Your anchor leg should be in a ninety-degree angle. Keep your hips, heels, and knees forward and aligned. Repeat, but step your left leg back. That's one rep. Perform fifteen reps (or fifteen lunges on each side).

3

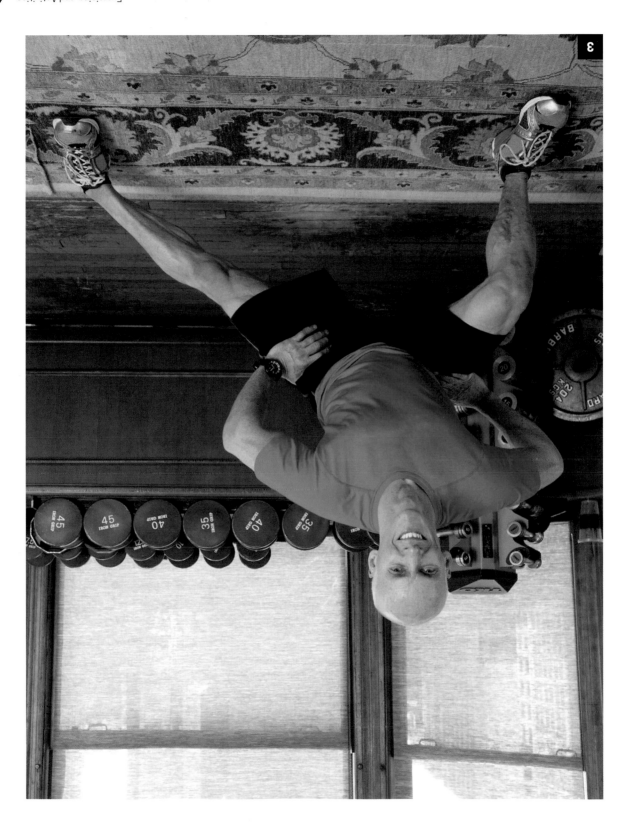

Switch Lunges

This challenging plyometric exercise is sure to blast your legs and glutes, while revving up your heart rate and boosting your metabolism.

1 Stand with your feet under your hips. Take a large step forward with your right foot. Sink down into a lunge, forming right angles with both legs.

2 Spring upward (2a), launching both feet off the floor, and switch positions with your legs so your left foot is in front and your right leg is behind (2b). Land and sink down into another lunge (2c). Alternate your legs (2d), completing fifteen repetitions on each side.

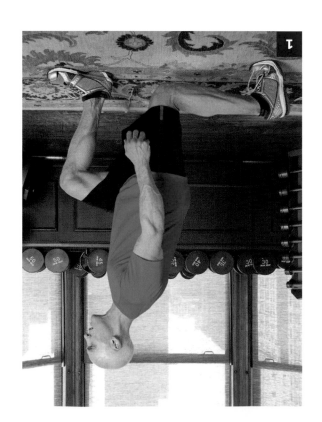

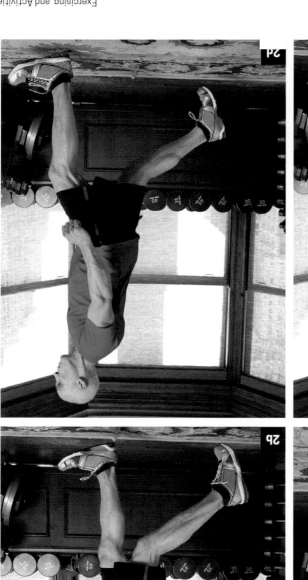

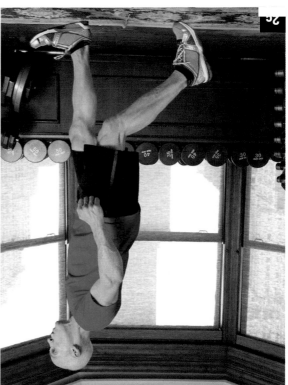

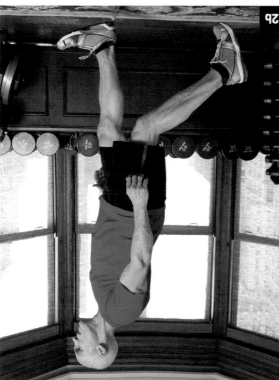

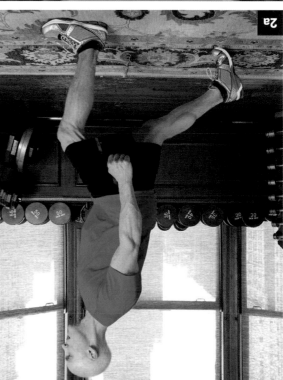

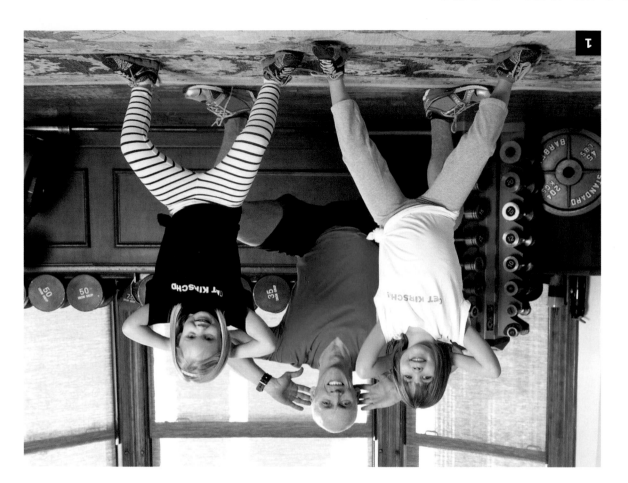

Platypus Walks

This is one of my favorite signature moves. You may look and feel silly while doing it, but if you nail the form, you will target your inner thighs and the lower half of your butt. You can see that Emilia and Francesca get a kick out of doing it too!

1 Start in a plié squat position with your hands on your hips and your thighs parallel to the floor.

2 Stay engaged in the plié squat as you waddle forward, stepping the left foot in front of the right, then the right foot in front of the left. Keep your knees out and aligned with your toes, your weight on your heels, and your butt sticking down and out throughout the exercise. Take five total steps forward, then reverse. That's one rep. Repeat five times.

2

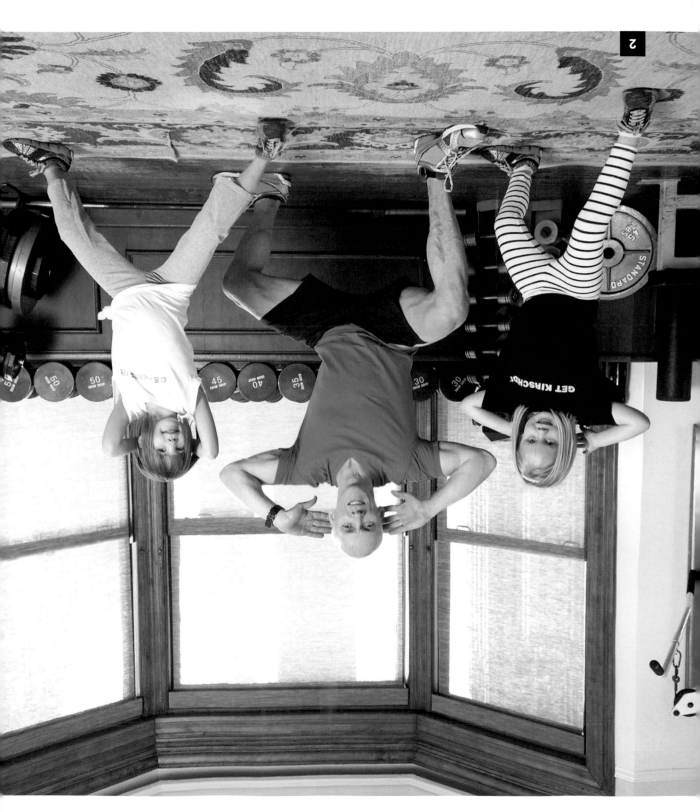

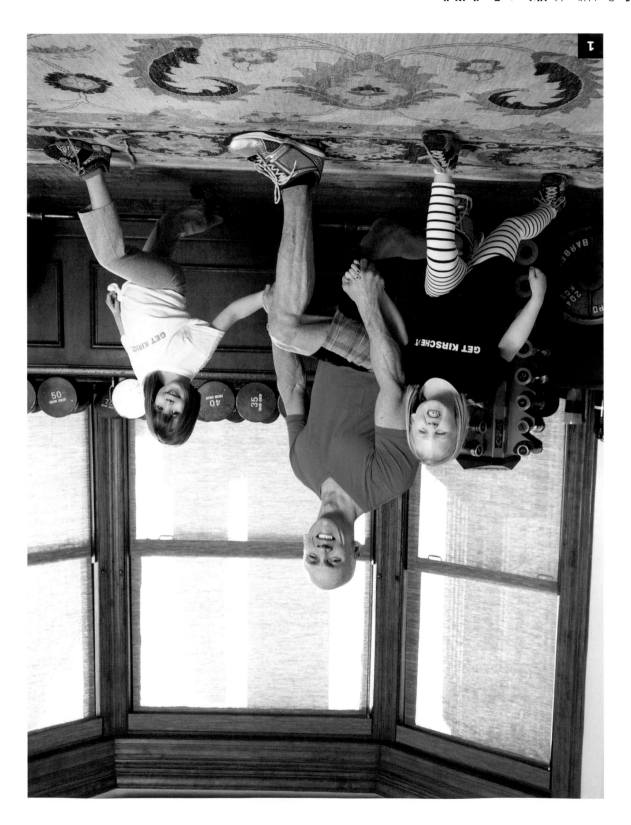

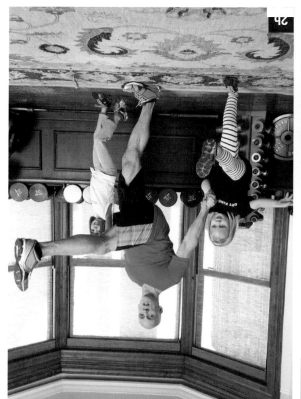

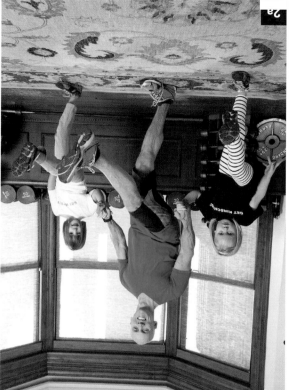

Reverse Lunge to High Kick

Are you getting ready to audition for The Rockettes? This is your move.

1 Stand with your feet shoulder-width apart with your hands on your hips. Take a large step back with your left foot, lunging so that both legs are bent in ninety-degree angles. (If you have problems with your knees, modify the degree at which you lunge. Partial ROM is safe and effective.) Additionally, I like to lean slightly forward in my lunge, placing more emphasis on my glutes.

2 Bring your right leg forward (2a) and go directly into a straight-leg high kick. Perform fifteen repetitions on each side.

Stability Ball Scissors

This exercise, one of my favorites to tighten and perk up your butt, is particularly good before hitting the beach or donning a fitted dress or pair of skinny jeans.

1 Lie face down on top of a stability ball with your hands on the floor close to the ball and your feet flexed and spread wide touching the ground.

2 Balance on your hands (2a) and then lift your legs and bring together your heels (2b), scissoring with your legs. Pause for five seconds (2c) then repeat. Do this fifteen times.

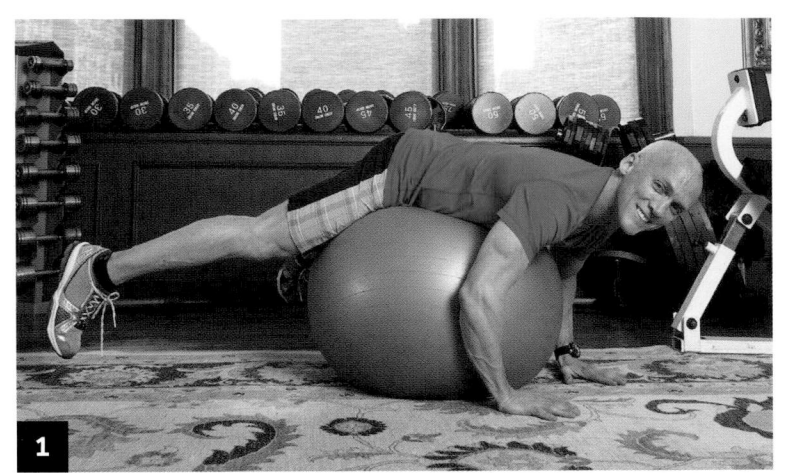

1

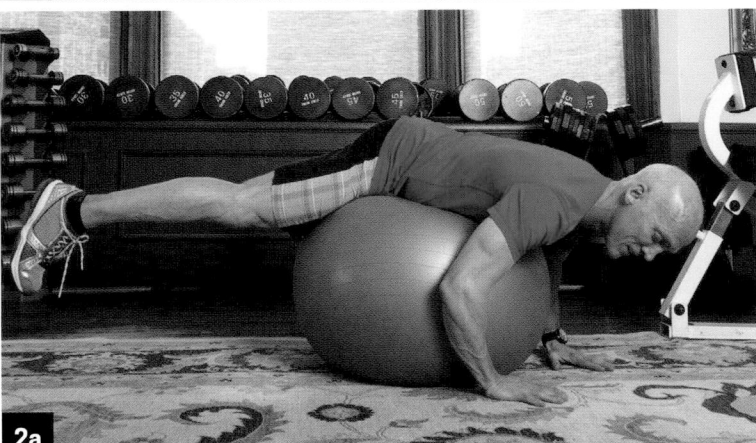

2a

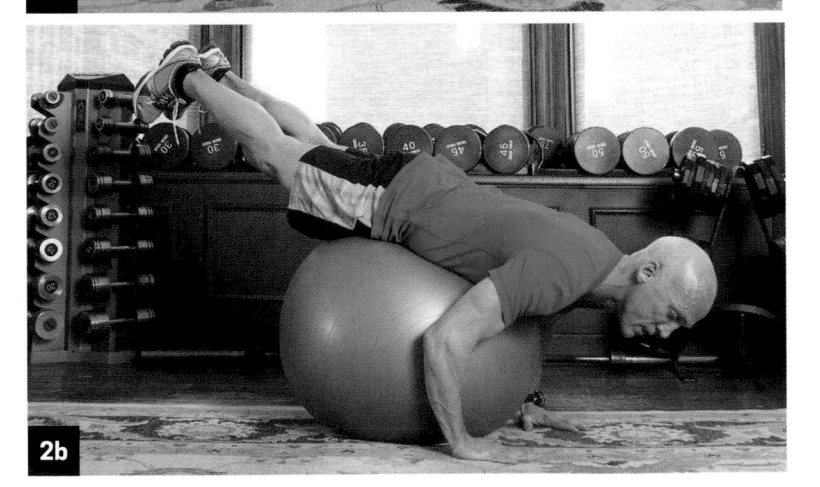

2b

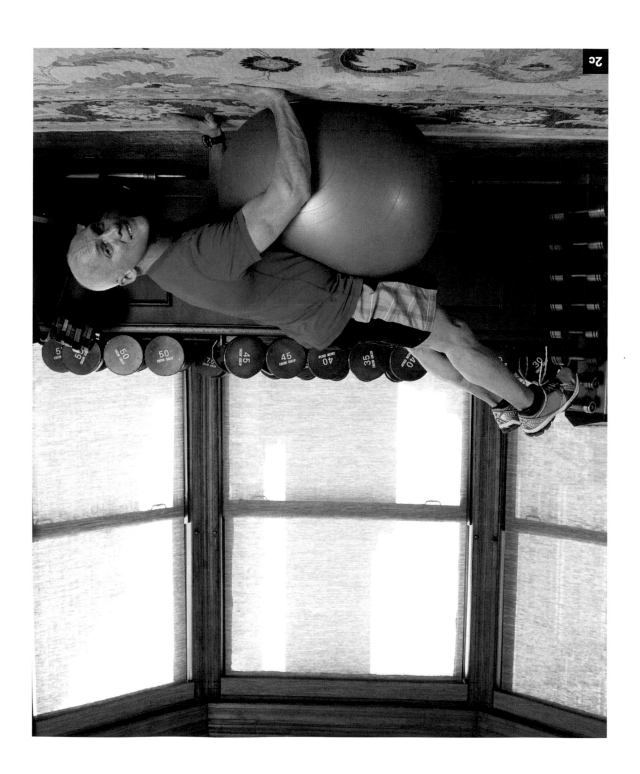

2c

Single-Leg Bridges on a Medicine Ball

Take your butt blast to the next level with this exercise.

1 Lie with your back flat on the floor. Place your heels on top of the medicine ball. Rest your hands about ninety degrees away from your sides with your palms facing down.

2 Press your right foot atop the medicine ball and lift your left leg straight up. Lift your hips toward the ceiling until only your head, shoulders, and arms touch the floor. Repeat fifteen times, then switch to the left leg and repeat fifteen more times. Make sure to engage your core and glutes throughout the exercise.

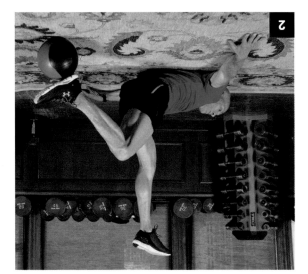

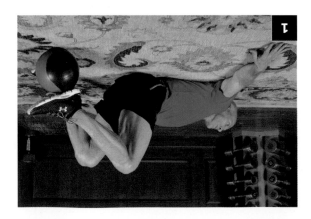

Jump Squats

This is another one of my go-to moves when I need a break from writing. It is a multipurpose exercise: It's a great plyometric move that I combine with other exercises, it clears my head, and it gets my heart pumping, all with the added bonus of strengthening, toning, and shaping. It is also a fun exercise to do with your kids.

1 Stand with your feet slightly wider than shoulder-width apart. Squat down and stick out your butt, making sure to keep your knees just above—not in front of—your toes.

2 Spring up and thrust your arms overhead. Tap your heels together and then bring your feet apart before you land on your heels, rolling forward on to your toes. Complete fifteen repetitions.

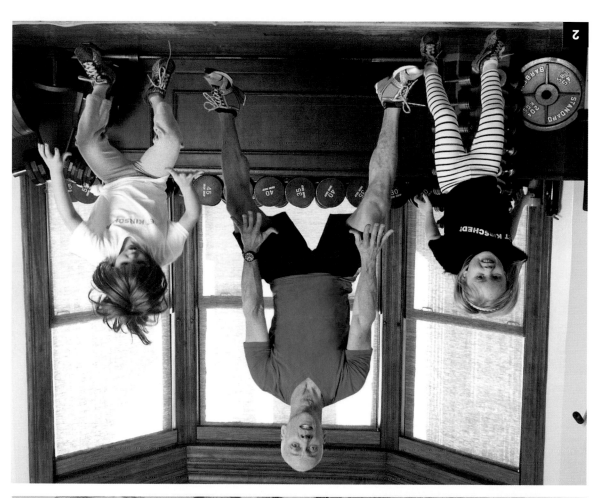

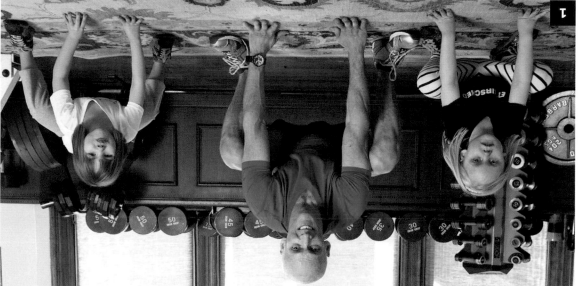

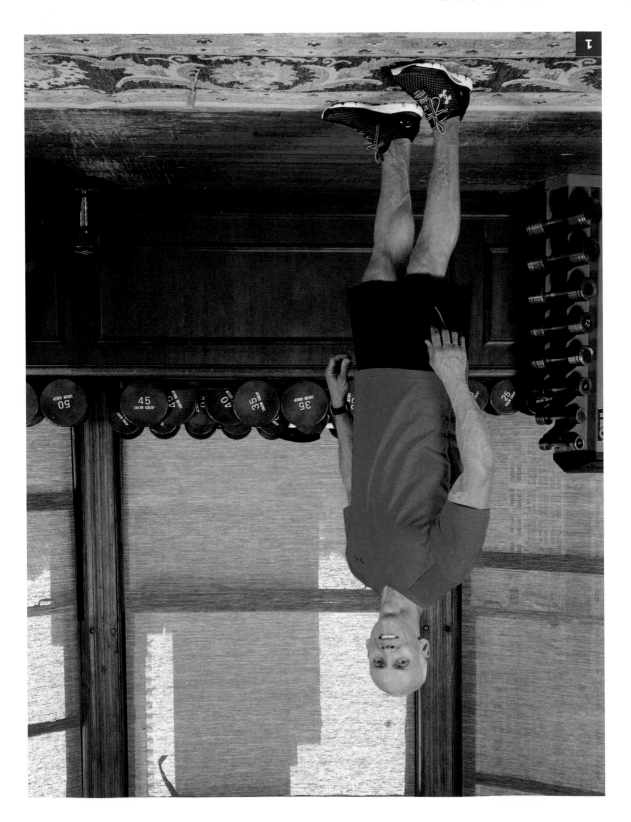

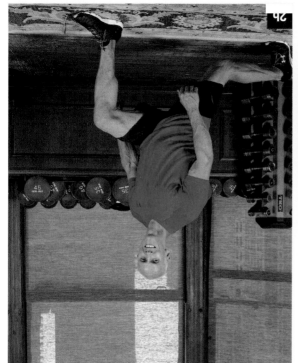

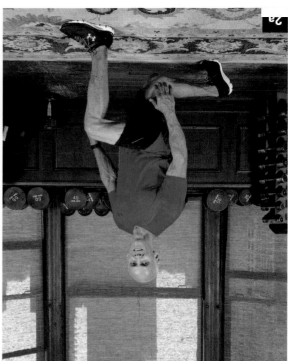

Forward and Reverse Lunges

Lunge, lunge, lunge away. Shape, tone, and sculpt your thighs and glutes being ever so mindful to keep your brain *where?* In your butt.

1 Stand with your feet shoulder-width apart.

2 Step your right foot forward into a lunge, landing on your right heel (2a). Bring your right leg back, stepping into the ball of your right foot, anchoring in your left heel (a reverse lunge) (2b),

and moving directly from the forward lunge so you never step down in the center. Perform fifteen repetitions and then switch legs and perform fifteen more.

Single-Leg Squat with a Stability Ball

This exercise may seem easy, but don't be fooled. Remember, the stability ball is anything but stable.

1 Stand with the stability ball about 12 inches (30.5 cm) behind your right leg. Bend your right knee and place the ball of your right foot on top of the stability ball.

2 Bend your left knee as you simultaneously straighten your right leg, pressing the stability ball back behind you.

3 Rise to the starting position and perform fifteen repetitions and then switch legs and perform fifteen more.

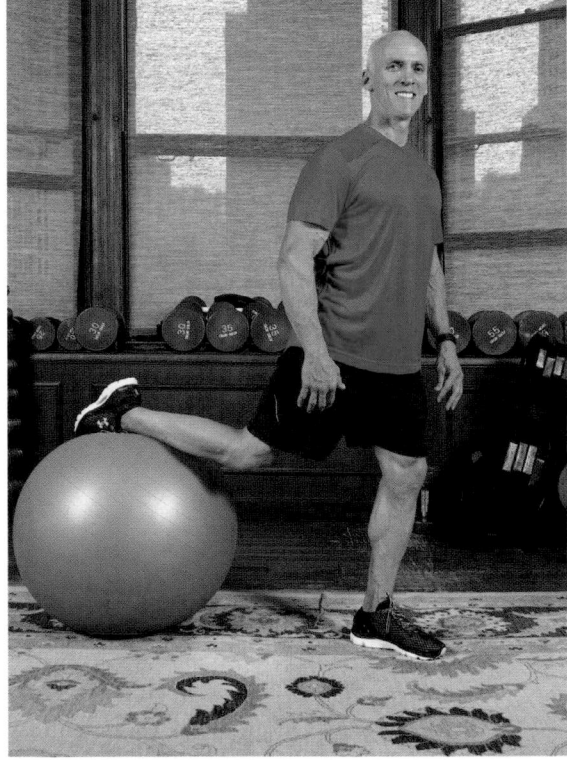
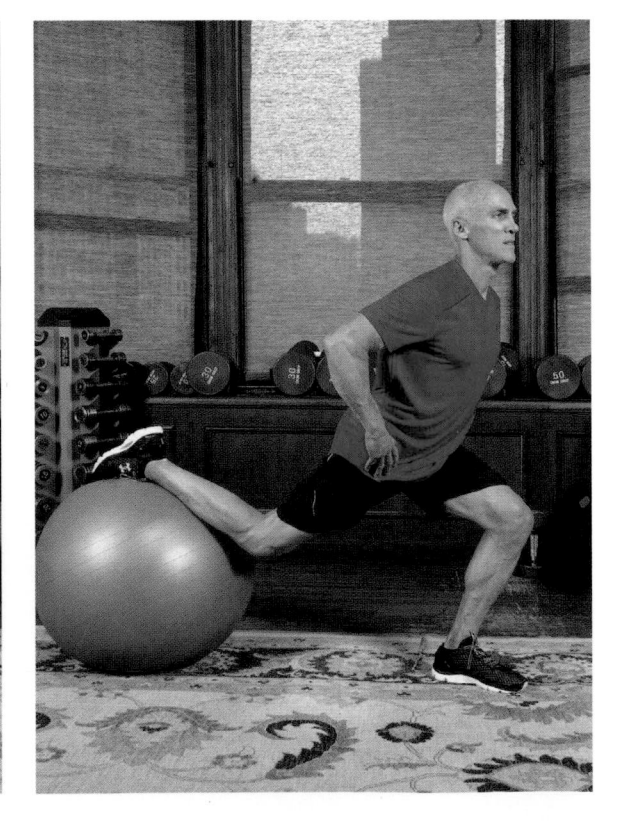

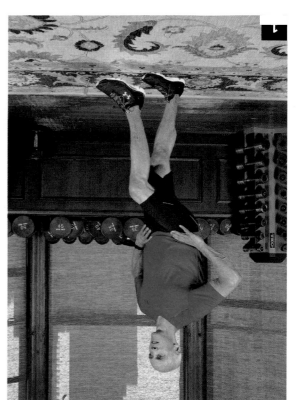

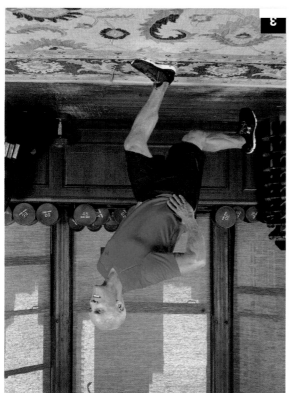

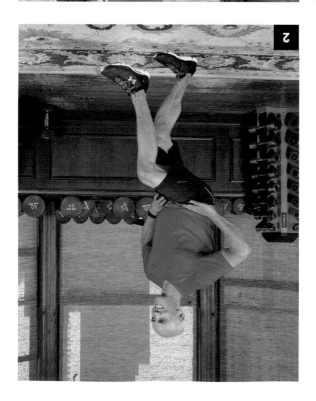

One-Legged Squats into Seesaws

This is a great exercise to do at home, in the office, or on vacation. It is particularly effective for engaging your quads, hamstrings, and glutes, especially if you don't have access to a gym or a stability ball.

1 Stand on one leg and bring the opposite knee up to a right angle.

2 Squat down so that your thigh is parallel to the floor.

3 Bring the raised knee back, extending the leg parallel to the floor. Do fifteen repetitions on each leg.

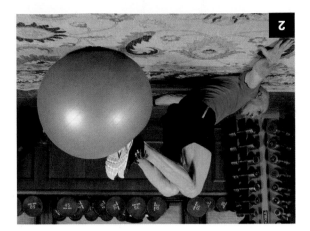

2

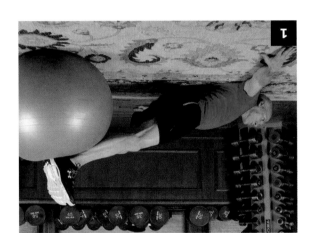

1

Hamstring Curls with a Stability Ball

For this exercise, choose from option A (the easier version) or option B (the more challenging version). To get into the bridge position, lie with your back on the floor and place your heels on top of the stability ball. Rest your hands about 90 degrees away from your sides with your palms facing down.

1 Option A: From the bridge position, lift your hips up off of the floor contracting your glutes. Slowly return to bridge position. Do fifteen repetitions.

2 Option B: From the bridge position, lift your hips up and simultaneously bend your knees and pull the ball in toward your butt. Push the ball back out into the bridge position. Do fifteen repetitions on each leg.

Bridge Position

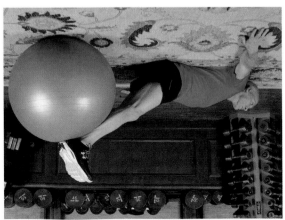

Lateral Lunge to a Hip Abduction

The hip abduction here not only works your inner thighs on the lateral movement, but also your outer thighs as you return to the starting position.

1 Start with your feet shoulder-width apart and your hands on your hips.

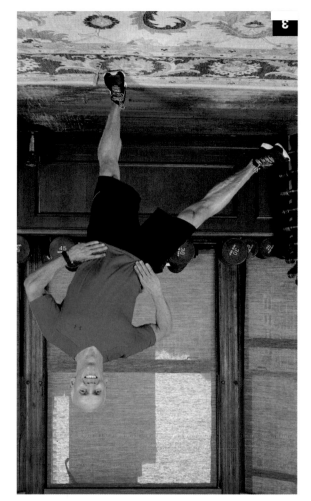

2 Step your right leg out to the side laterally. Make sure to step into your right heel, keeping the right knee aligned with your right heel. Your anchor leg should be held straight in a ninety-degree angle. Keep your hips, heels, and knees forward and aligned.

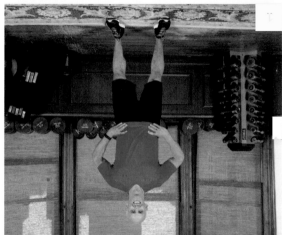

3 Return to the starting position and immediately lift your left leg out laterally, keeping your foot flexed and your left heel off the ground (i.e., hip abduction). Do fifteen repetitions on each leg.

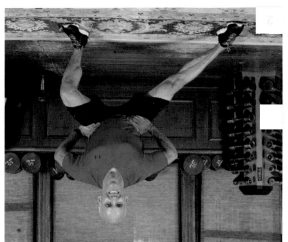

UPPER BODY EXERCISES (Back, Torso, and Arms)

These exercises are designed for people who wear baggy tops and sweaters to hide the weight they carry in their bellies, back, and arms. Though you may be able to mask extra fat that you think unsightly, you can't hide from the fact that carrying that extra weight is unhealthy, especially so near to your heart.

These circuits attack your trouble spots and even out your physique. To get the most from the movements, avoid engaging your shoulders and traps as much as possible. Instead, work hard to engage your core and maintain proper postural alignment (see the sidebar "Good Form Means Great Results," page 32). Visualize what you're doing and the results you want.

Jumping Jacks with Shoulder Presses

This exercise brings me back to my high school Phys Ed class. It's a great exercise for arms, shoulders, and core.

1 Stand with your feet under your hips. Grasp a dumbbell in each hand (or a water bottle if you don't have dumbbells) with your elbows bent and hands at ear height.

2 Jump your feet out into a wide angle as you press the dumbbells overhead, keeping them above your shoulders. Bring your feet back together as you lower the dumbbells. Repeat thirty times.

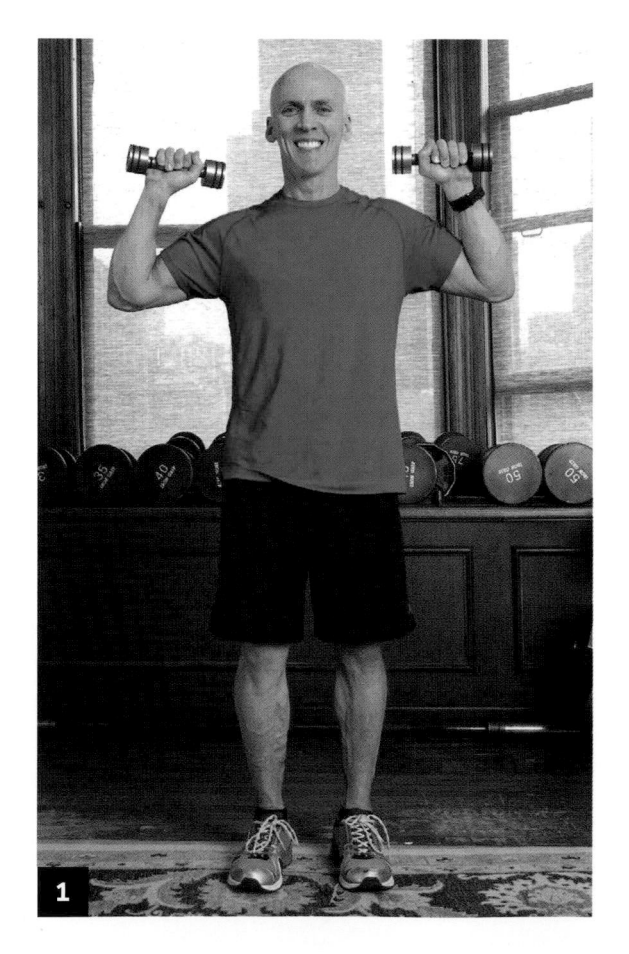

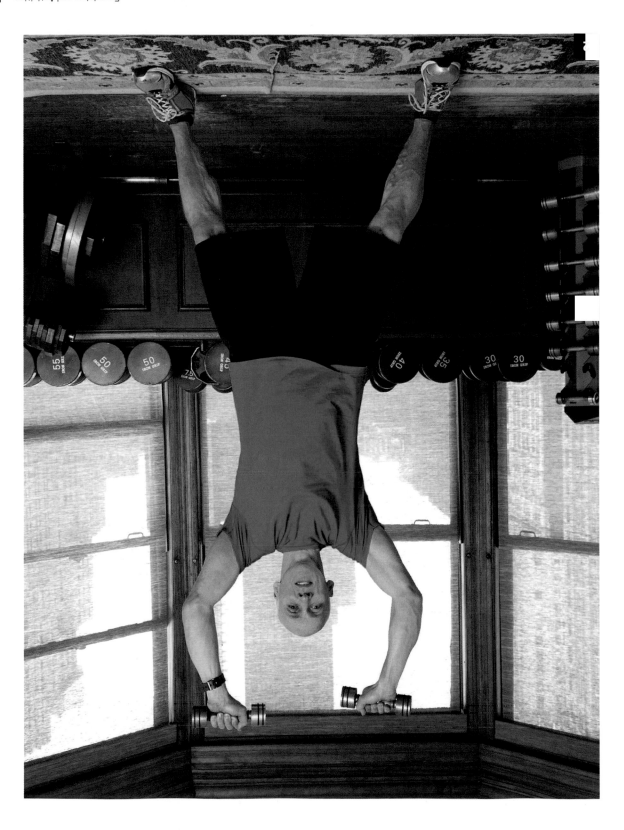

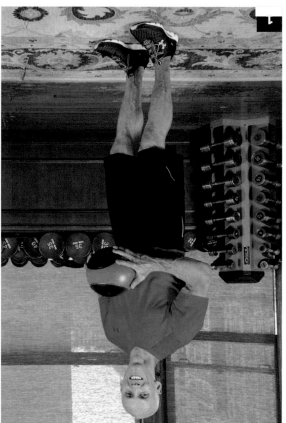

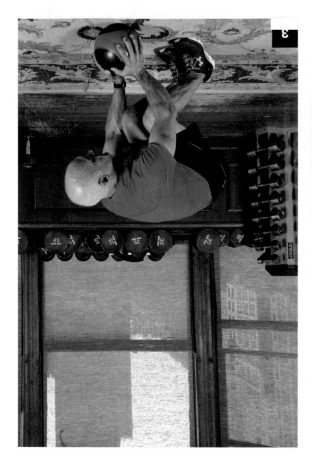

Burpees with a Medicine Ball

As if burpees weren't challenging enough, let's do them while balancing on a medicine ball.

1 Stand with your feet slightly wider than hip-width apart. Grasp a medicine ball with both hands at chest level with your elbows bent.

2 Bend your knees, stick your butt back, and move into a squat position.

3 Continue to bend your knees as you bend forward from the hips, placing the medicine ball on the floor under your chest.

4 Press your hands into the medicine ball as you jump and extend your legs behind your body, progressing into a plank position. Keep your core engaged the entire time. Recoil your legs and rise to the starting position. Do fifteen repetitions.

5 During your final repetition, remain in the plank position and proceed directly into Mountain Climbers (described next).

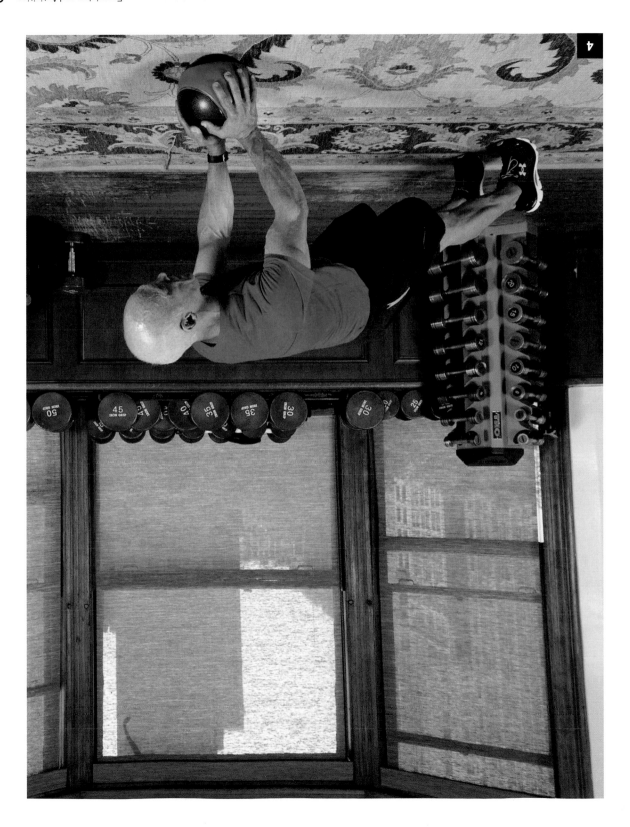

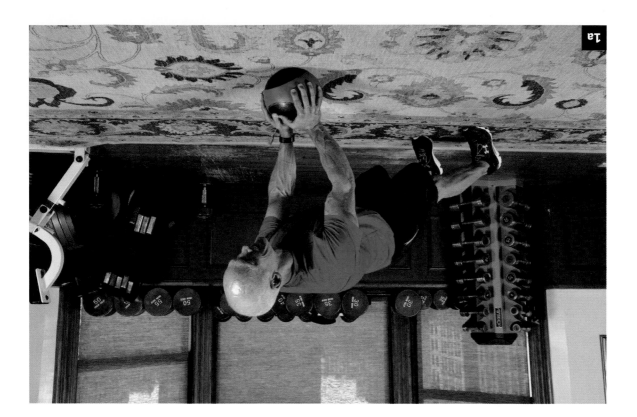

Mountain Climbers with a Medicine Ball

Immediately following your final Burpee, balance over the ball, keep your core engaged, and visualize the core and body of your dreams. This exercise requires strength, balance, and coordination.

1 From the plank position of your final Burpee (1a), bend your right knee and jump it in, bringing your right thigh under the right side of your torso (1b).

2 Jump your right leg back as you simultaneously bend your left knee and jump it in. Continue alternating right and left for thirty seconds.

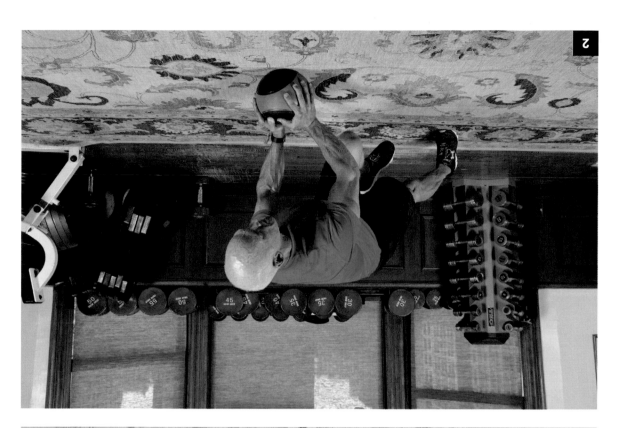

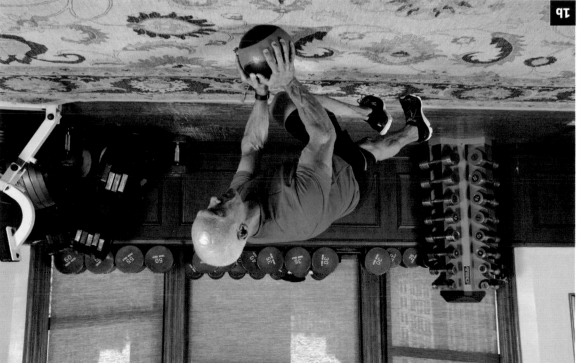

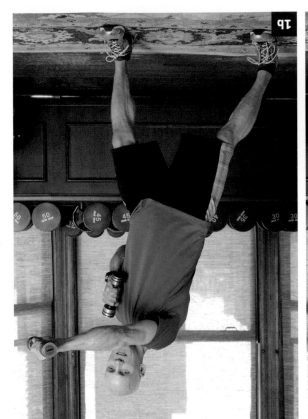

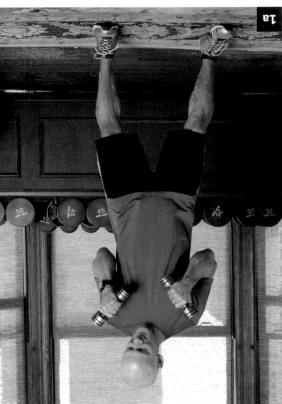

Shadow Boxing

This is a great way to de-stress while shaping your arms, back, and shoulders.

1 Grasp a dumbbell (or a water bottle) in each hand. Stand with your abs tight and your back flat (1a). Punch your left fist out diagonally, ending at torso level in front of your ribs, completing a crossover punch. Pull back as you bend your knees, as if ducking an incoming punch. Repeat on the other side as you extend your legs, driving up from your heels and into your butt. Do thirty repetitions with each arm.

2 With your left elbow against your ribs and your knuckles turned up, punch upward as if punching someone in the jaw under the chin with an uppercut, trying to lift him or her off the ground. Pull back as you bend your knees, sitting back on your heels. Do thirty repetitions on each side.

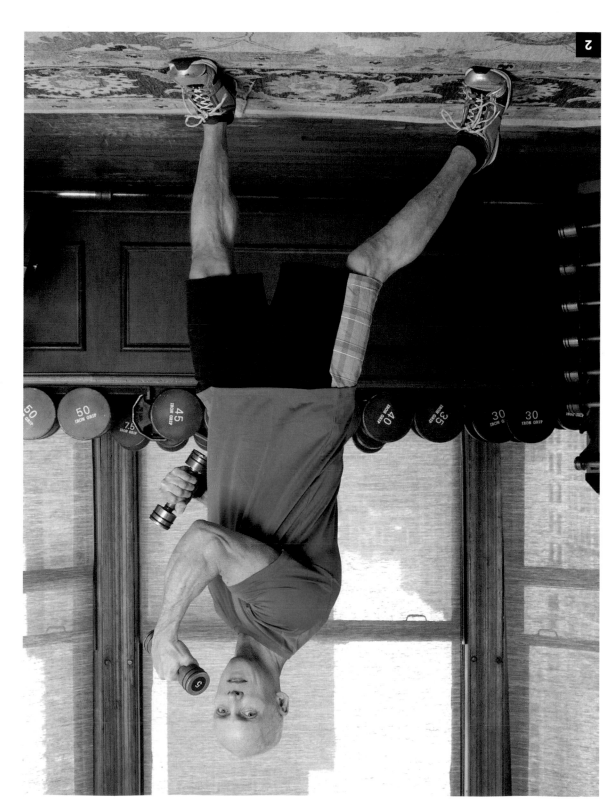

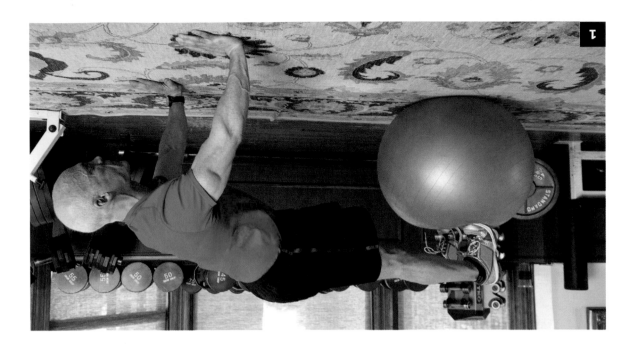

1.

Stability Ball Pushups to Knee Tuck

Targeting the chest, upper back, arms, and core, this exercise will challenge you and deliver real results quickly.

1 Place your tummy on the stability ball and palms on the floor in front of the ball. Walk your hands forward as you slide your torso forward on the ball, until you come into a pushup position with your thighs, shins or balls of your feet on the ball. (Note: Placing your thighs on the ball is the least challenging option, your shins slightly more challenging, and the balls of your feet or your toes the most challenging.) Place your palms on the floor under your chest. Make sure your abs are tight and back is flat. Do not allow your hips to sink downward.

2 Bend your elbows out to the sides as your lower your chest toward the floor. Exhale as you extend your elbows and push up to the starting position.

3 From the pushup position, bend your knees and bring them in toward your chest. Extend your legs as you push the ball back to the starting position. Keep your abs tight the entire time.

4 From a pushup position with the balls of your feet on the stability ball, raise your hips toward the ceiling as you bring the ball in towards your hands, keeping your abs tight and legs extending. Your torso should form an upside down V shape. Hold for 5 seconds.

Proceed back to the pushups, knee tucks and pike combination 10–15 repetitions.

NOTE: When you've mastered this move, try dialing up the intensity by placing your hands closely together in a diamond shape. (See photo on page 78.) This will give added focus to your triceps and core!

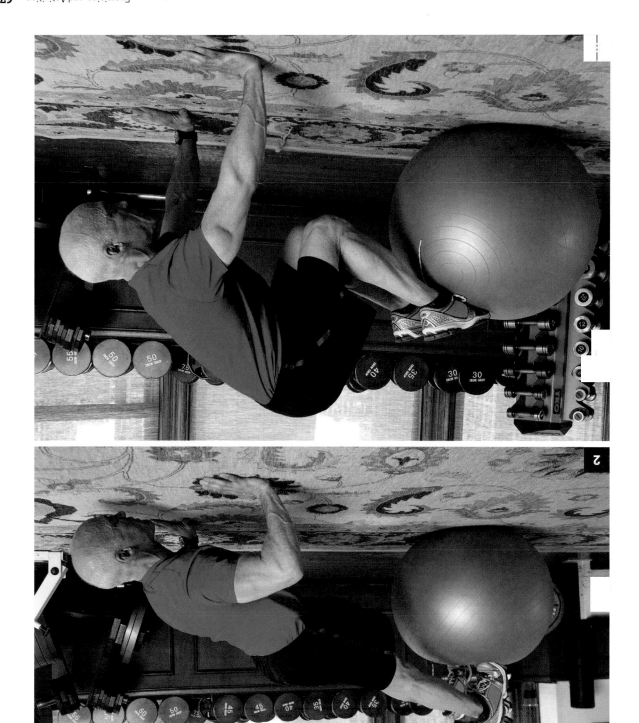

2

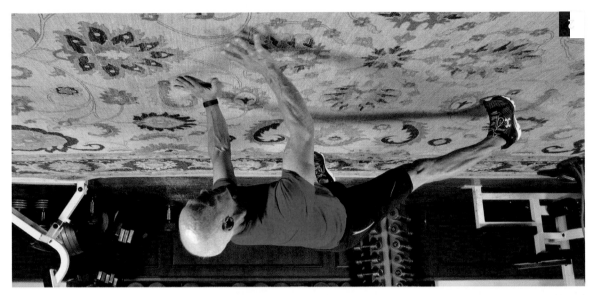

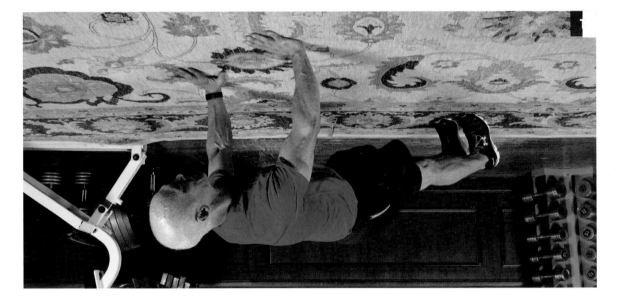

Walking Planks

This exercise is a simple and effective twist for your core and arms.

1 Start in a plank position on your hands and toes.

2 Walk your body five steps to the left and then five steps back to center. That's one repetition. Repeat five times on each side.

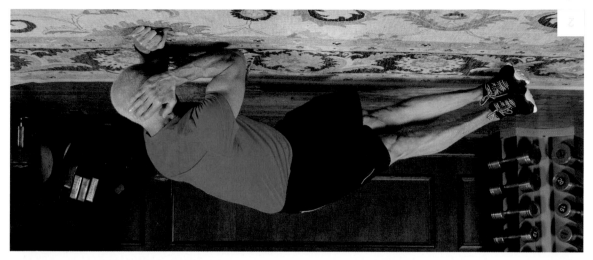

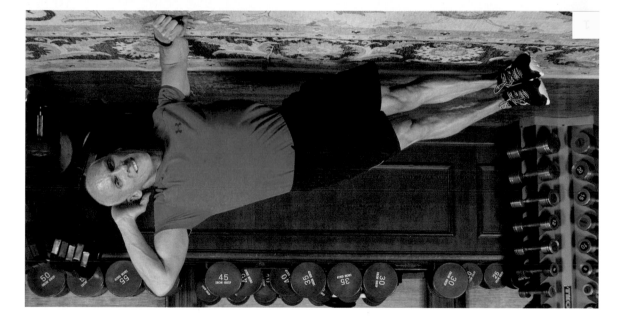

Side Plank Oblique Crunches

Kiss your love handles goodbye.

1 Position yourself in a side plank, resting on your right forearm with your left arm behind your head.

2 Bring your left elbow in toward your belly and then return to the starting position. Perform fifteen repetitions on each side.

Plank with Torso Rotation to T-Stand

Raise the level on your plank by rotating your torso and extending your arm overhead, firing up your triceps and obliques.

1 Starting in a plank position and holding a dumbbell in your right hand (1a), reach your right arm under your torso (1b and 1c) and then back out, rotating your body to a side plank (1d) as your right arm extends straight up (your arm should form a "T" with your body).

2 That's one rep. Perform fifteen repetitions on each side.

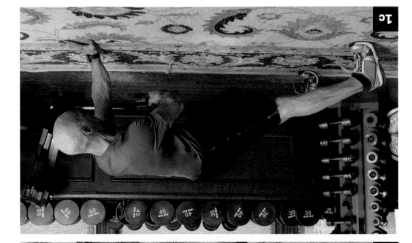

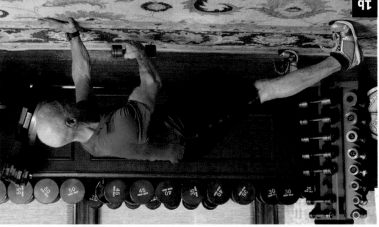

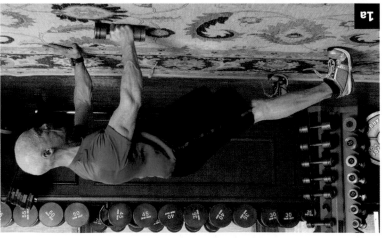

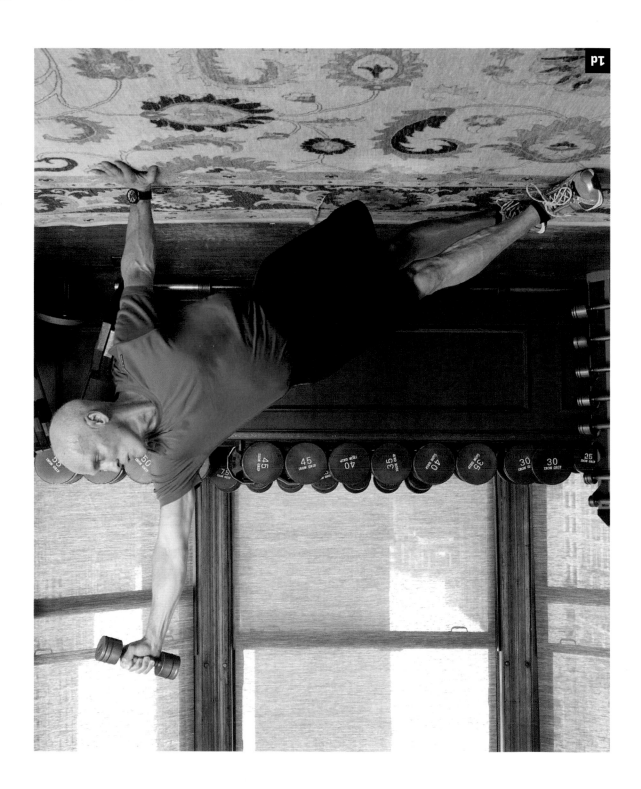

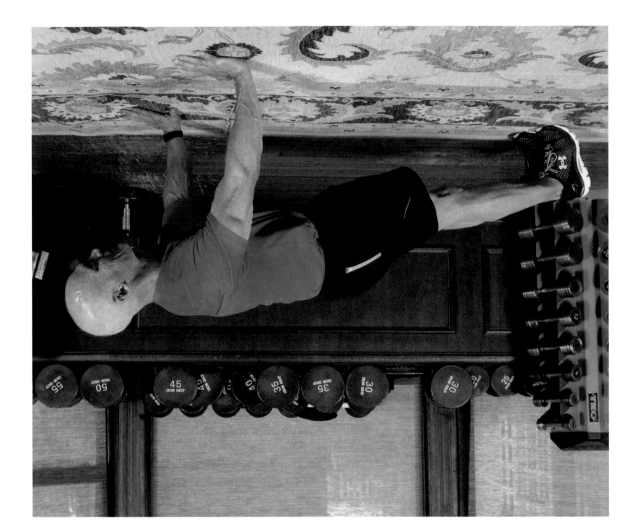

Pushups with a Hip Extension

Put a little twist in your pushup routine.

1 Get into a pushup position with your hands shoulder-width apart and directly under your chest.

2 Lower yourself into a pushup while simultaneously lifting your right leg 6 inches (15 cm) off the ground, keeping it straight and your foot flexed. Perform ten repetitions and then repeat with the other leg.

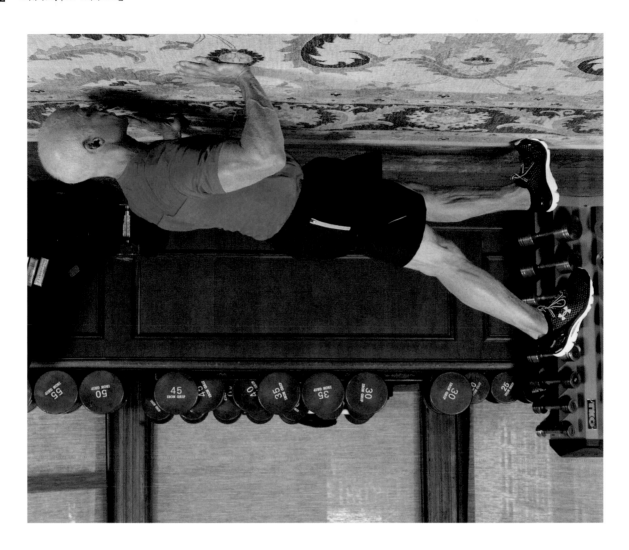

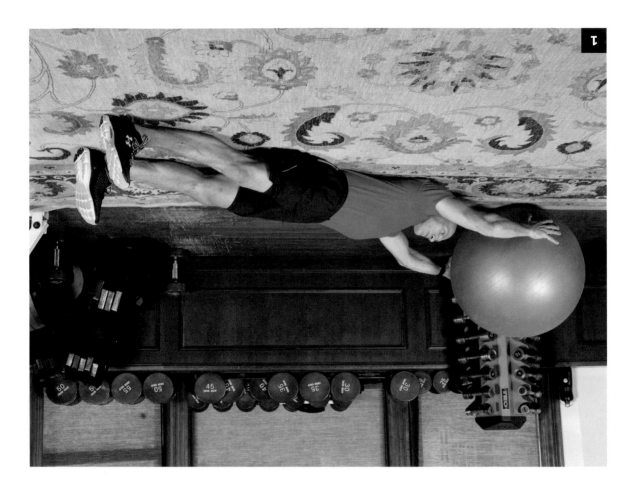

1

Stability Ball Handoffs

This is one of my favorite signature ab exercises. It really blasts the abs from every angle.

1 Lie flat on your back with a stability ball in your hands.

2 Lift your torso and your hands to meet your legs in the middle, pause, and pass the ball so you're now holding it between your legs.

3 Return to lying flat on your back, this time with the stability ball between your legs. Then lift your torso and legs again to meet and return the ball to your arms. Perform fifteen repetitions.

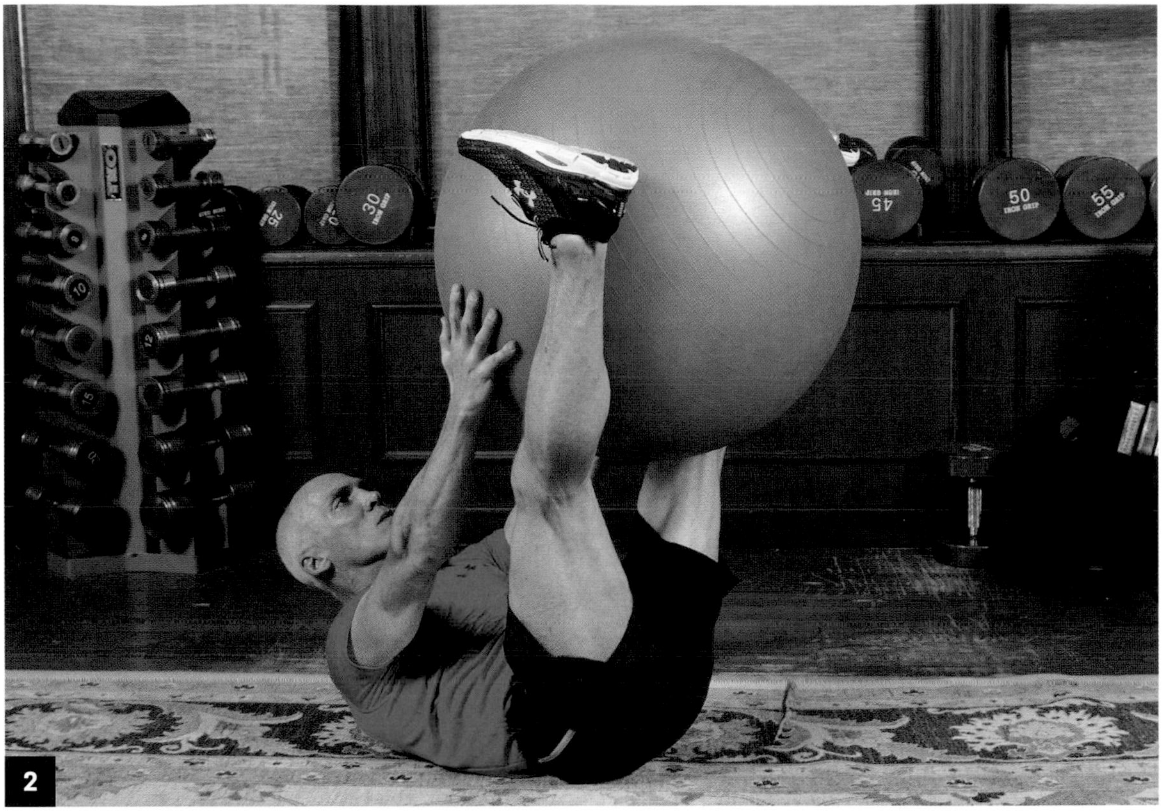

2

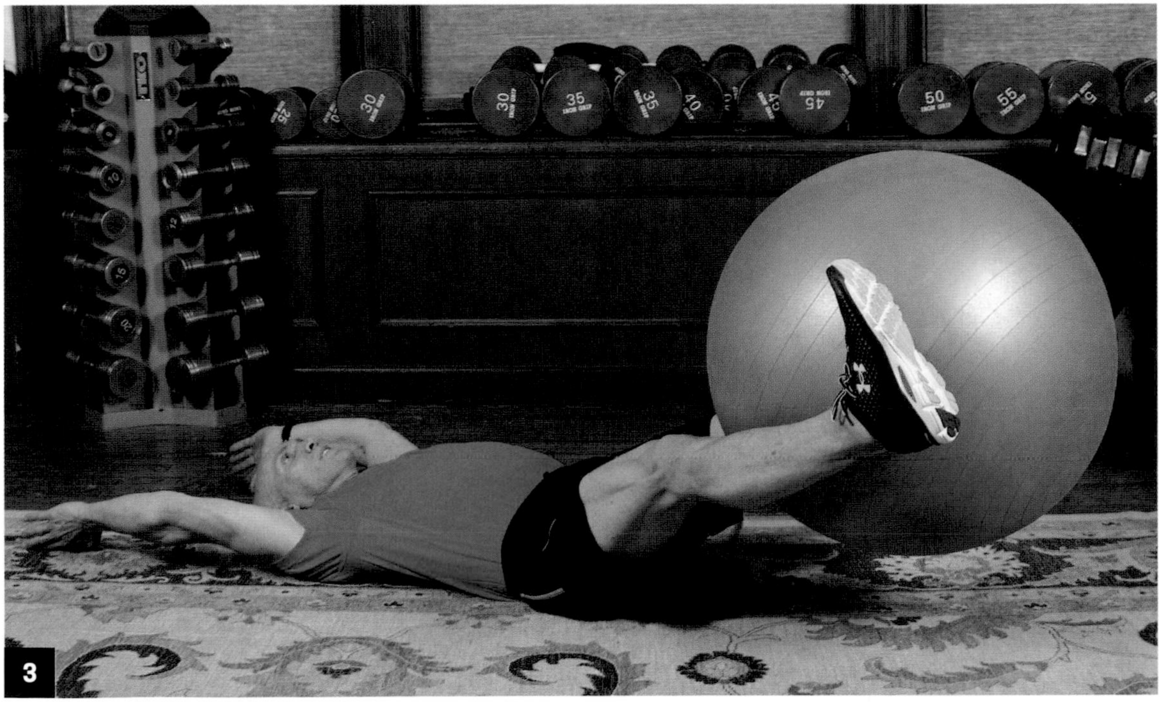

3

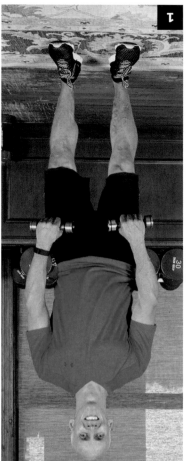

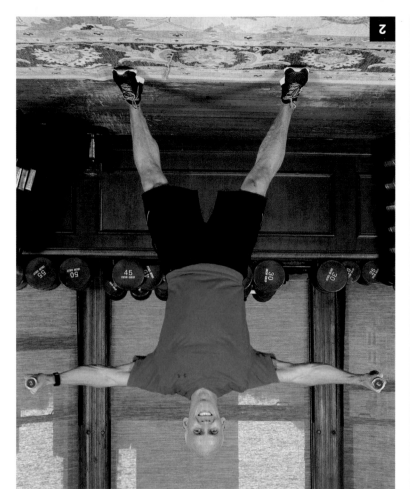

Jumping Jacks with Lateral and Front Raises

I love this twist on jumping jacks. It really fires up your shoulders and blasts your core.

1 Stand with your feet under your hips. Grasp a dumbbell (or water bottle) in each hand, holding your hands at your sides with your palms facing in.

2 Jump your feet out into a wide angle as you raise your arms out to your sides to shoulder height, palms facing down and parallel to the floor. Bring your feet back together as you lower your arms.

3 Jump your feet out into a wide angle as you raise your arms straight in front of you, palms facing down and parallel to the floor. Bring your feet back together as you lower your arms.

4 Alternate side and front laterals, fifteen repetitions each.

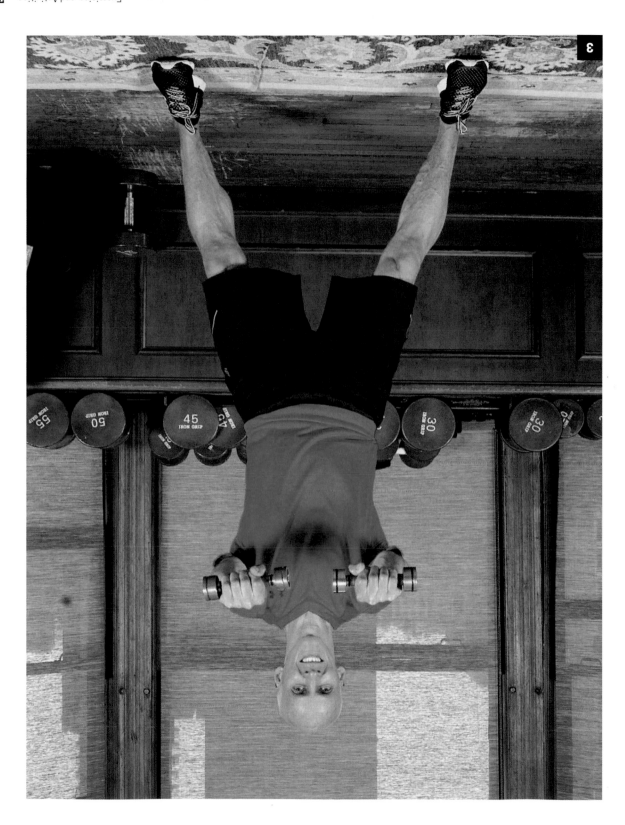

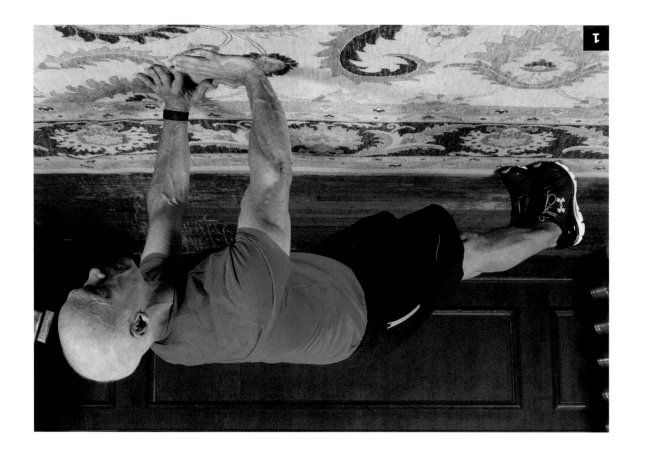

Diamond Pushups

This variation on pushups really turns up the dial on shaping your chest and blasting your triceps and core.

1 Place your hands close together so your thumbs and forefingers touch and form a diamond shape.

2 Lower yourself into a pushup position, making sure to keep your arms tucked in close to your sides. Return to the starting position. Do fifteen repetitions.

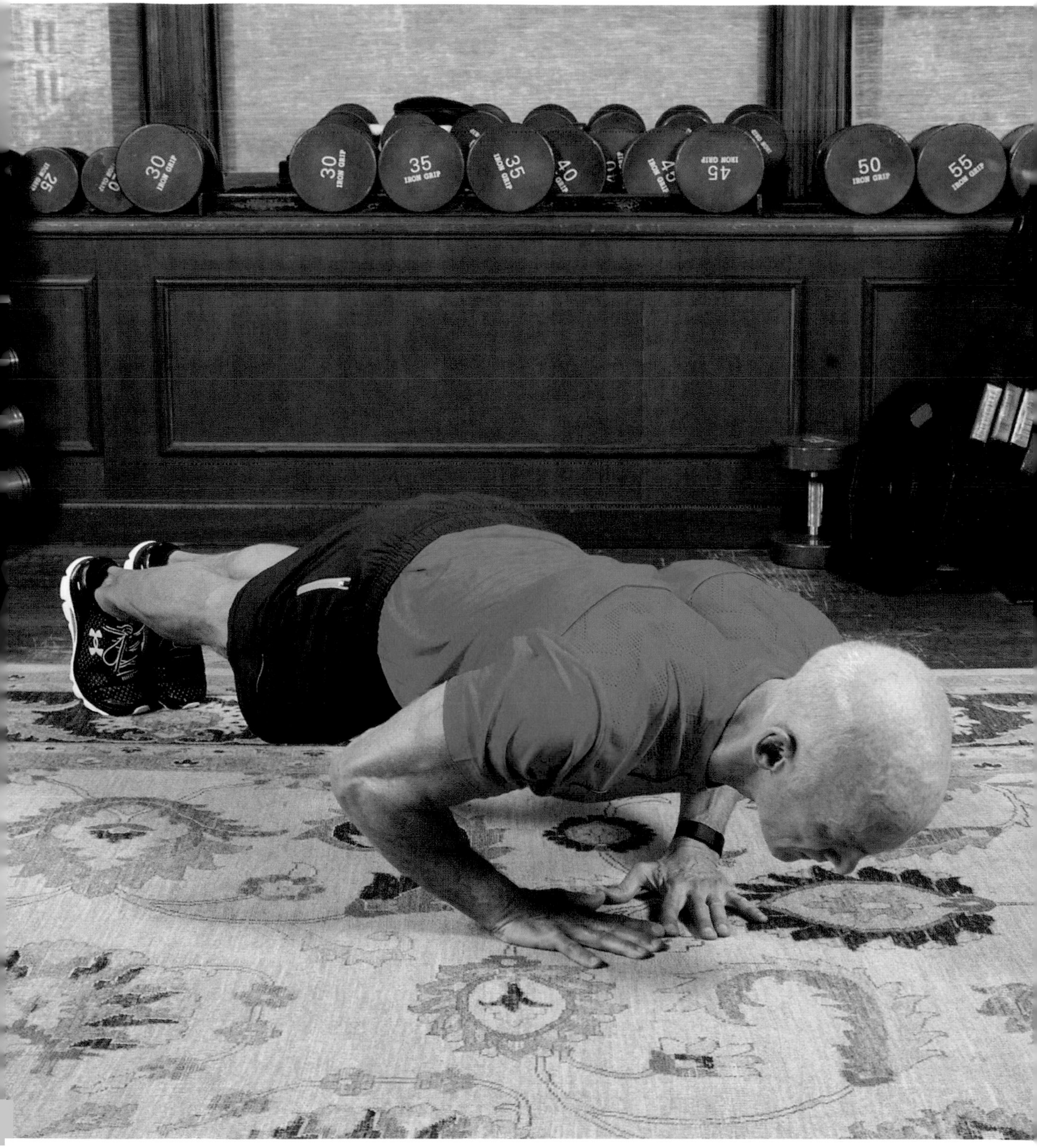
25
30
30
35
IRON GRIP
35
40
45
50
IRON GRIP
55

UPPER AND LOWER BODY EXERCISES

If you carry your weight more democratically over your whole body, you need to work your whole body.

These exercises use compound moments that engage your lower and upper body at the same time. If you're lunging with your lower body, you need to be moving some weight with your upper body. If you're working your back, you need to also work your butt and legs.

Around the World with a Medicine Ball

This signature move starts off feeling nice and easy, but halfway through, you'll see that you're engaging your arms, back, shoulders, hamstrings, and abs. In fact, they are being quietly and effectively blasted.

1 Stand with your feet shoulder-width apart. Hold a medicine ball extended overhead.

2 Bend to the side from your hips (2a) in a half circle down the right side of your body past your toes (2b) and up the left side of your body (2c) until the ball once again rests overhead. Repeat a half circle to your left. Continue circling right and left, fifteen repetitions in each direction.

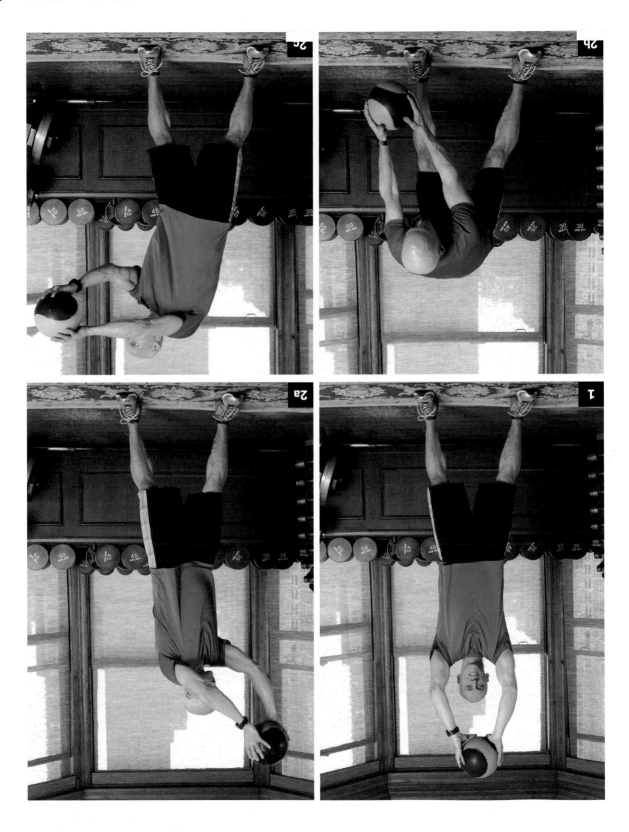

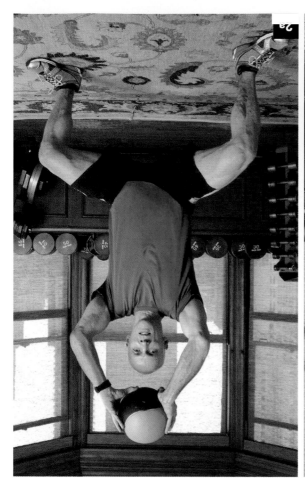

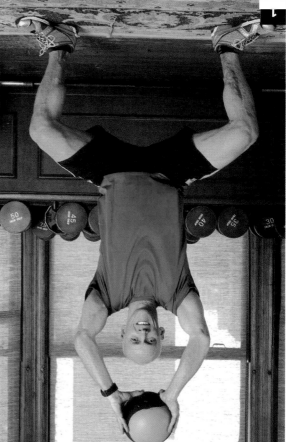

Platypus Walks with a Medicine Ball Overhead

Do you want to blast your core while you tone your butt and thighs?

Try this move.

1 Start in a plié squat position with your arms extended overhead and holding a medicine ball and with your thighs parallel to the floor.

2 Stay engaged in the plié squat as you waddle forward, stepping the left foot in front of the right, then the right foot in front of the left (2a). Keep your knees out and aligned with your toes, your weight in your heels, and your butt sticking down and out throughout the exercise (2b). Take five total steps forward and then reverse. That's one rep. Repeat five times.

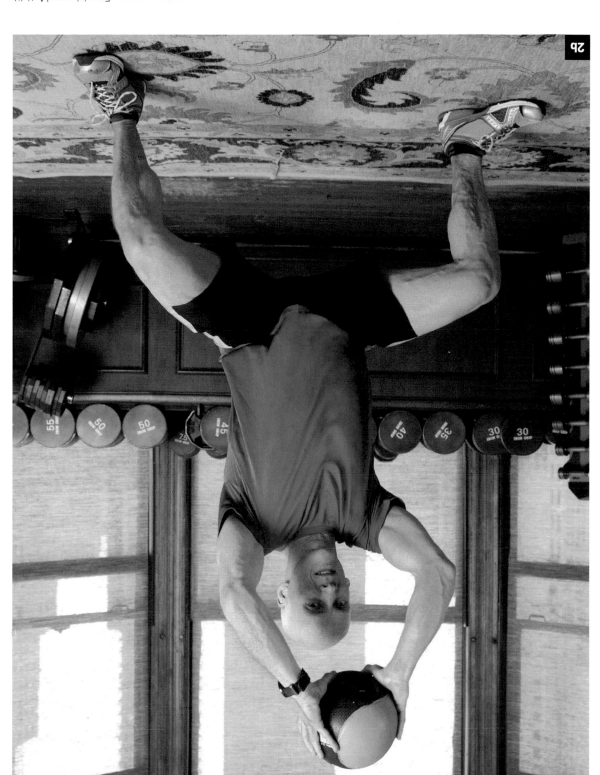

2b

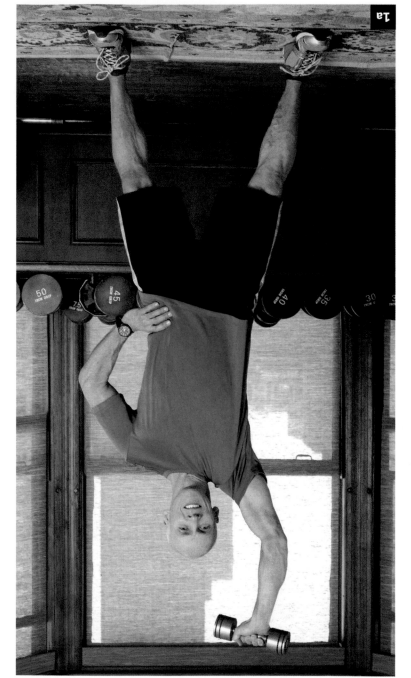

1a

Squat with One Dumbbell Overhead

Adding a single dumbbell overhead to your basic wide-stance squat helps engage and strengthen your core and legs.

1 Start with your feet shoulder-width apart, holding a dumbbell (or a water bottle) straight overhead in your right hand (1a). Complete fifteen squats (1b).

2 Switch the dumbbell to your left hand and do fifteen more.

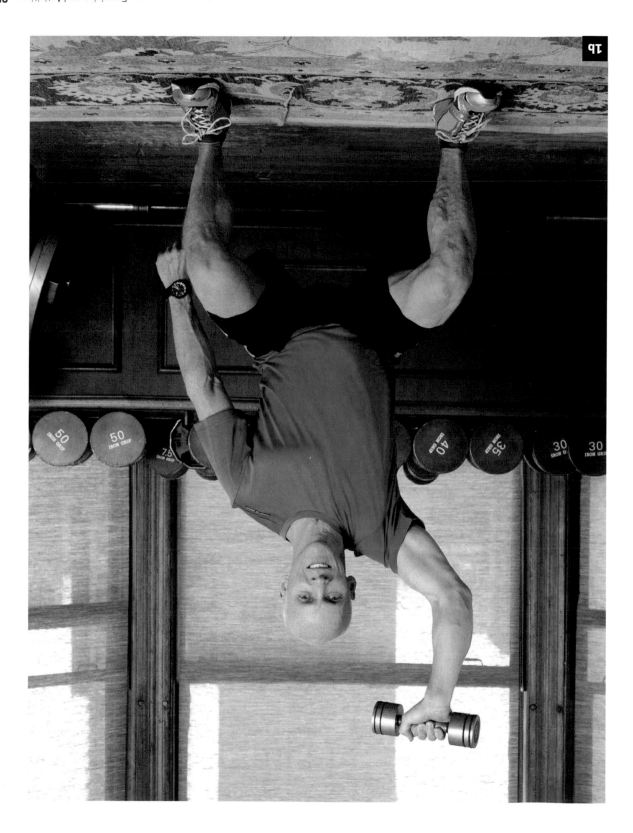

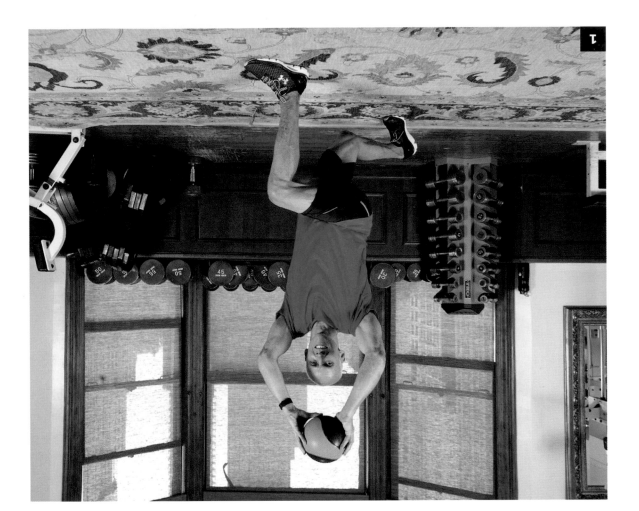

Switch Lunges with a Medicine Ball Overhead

If this exercise wasn't challenging enough, you're going to hold a medicine ball overhead for an extra core blast.

1 Stand in the "up" position of a lunge, with your right foot in front of your left and your arms extended, holding a medicine ball overhead.

2 Leap into the air, switching legs. Plant your front heel as you land in a lunge with your left leg forward. That's one repetition. Immediately leap back into the air. Continue switching sides and leaping until you complete fifteen lunges on each side.

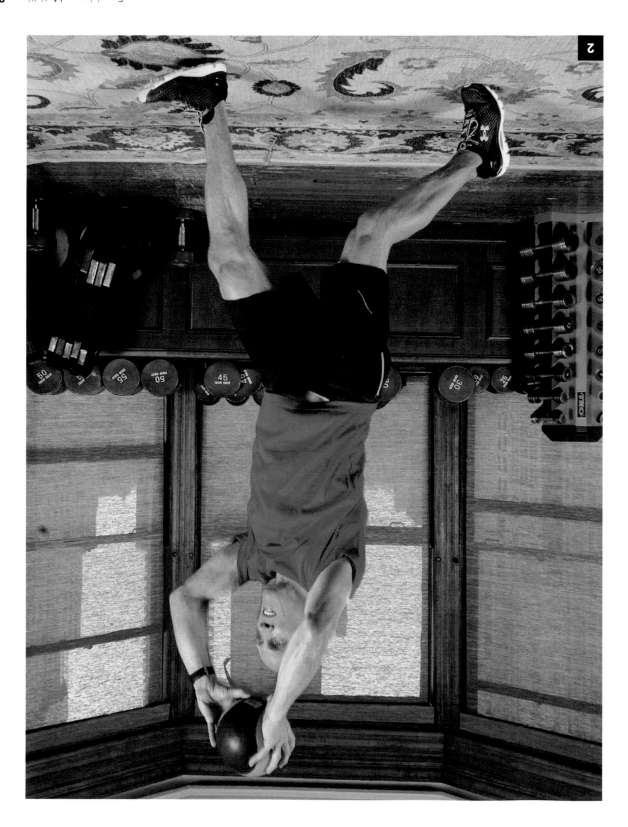

2

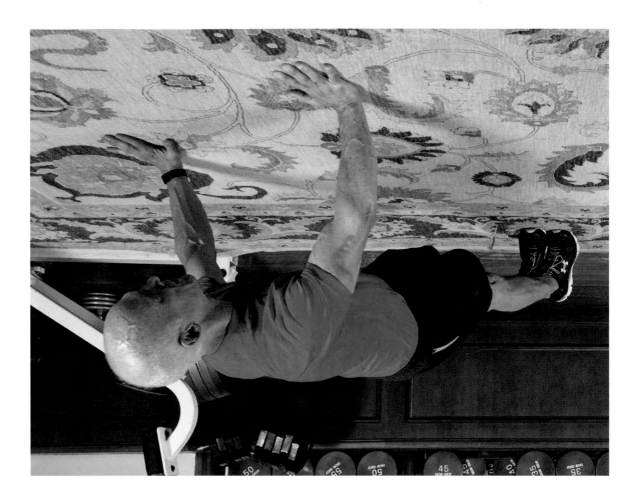

Wheelbarrow Planks

I saw this being done in a gym once, and I quickly incorporated and adapted it into my regimen. This takes the simple (yet challenging) plank to a whole new level.

1 Start in a plank position on your hands and toes.

2 Using your feet as the axis, maintain an engaged core and perfect plank as you rotate your body a full 360-degree circle counterclockwise and back to your starting position, then clockwise and back to your starting position. That's one repetition. Do two.

Medicine Ball Wood Chop to a Lateral Lunge

Engage your arms, core, thighs, and butt all at once with this exercise.

1 Start with your feet shoulder-width apart and a medicine ball in your arms, up and out to your right at eye level.

2 Simultaneously step out to the left into a lateral lunge while swinging the medicine ball across your body, pointing it toward the front of your left foot with straight arms. Do fifteen repetitions and then switch to the other side and do fifteen more.

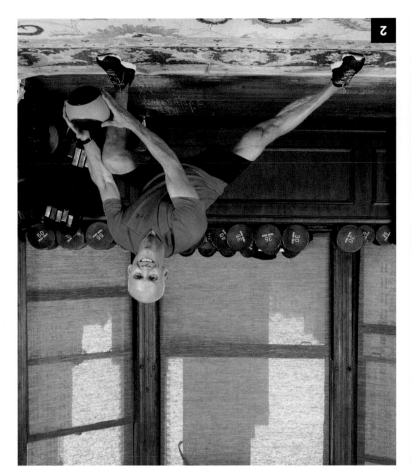

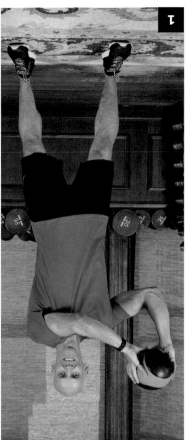

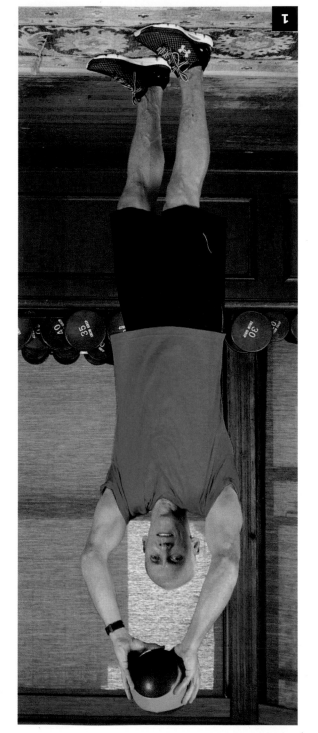

Forward and Reverse Lunge with a Medicine Ball Overhead

Adding the medicine ball overhead forces you to engage your core while you assault your legs and butt.

1 Stand with your feet shoulder-width apart, holding a medicine ball overhead.

2 Step your right foot forward into a lunge, landing on your right heel. Bring your right leg back to a reverse lunge, moving directly from the forward lunge so you never step down in the center. Do fifteen repetitions and then switch legs and do fifteen more.

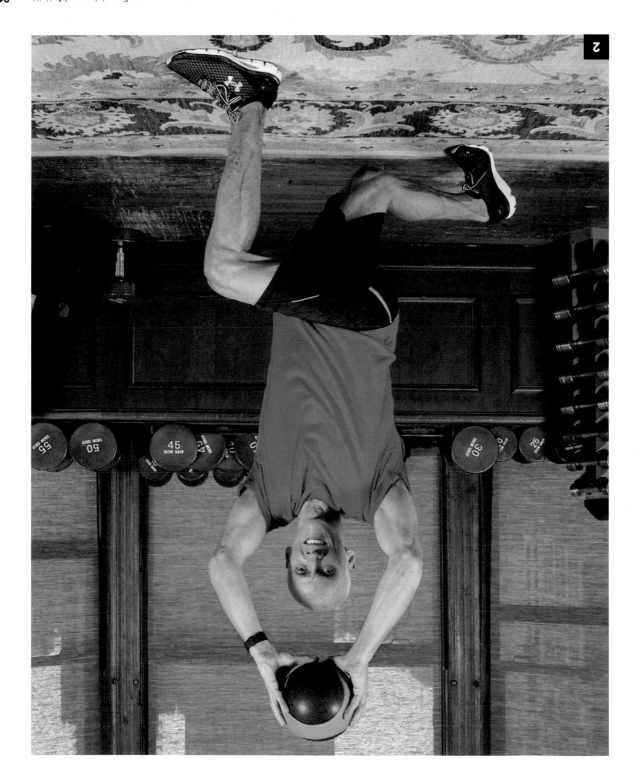

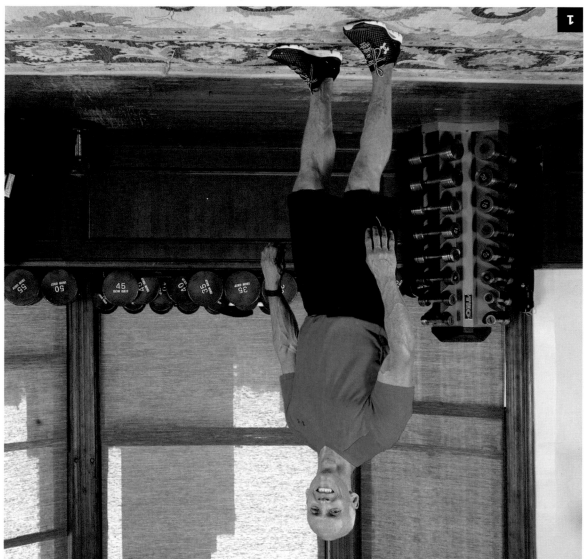

1.

Burpees with Spiderman Pushups

This exercise is a total-body blast.

1 Stand with your feet shoulder-width apart.

2 Place your hands on the floor and quickly kick your legs straight out behind you.

3 Lower yourself into a pushup, then bring your right knee toward your right shoulder. During the next pushup, bring your left knee toward your left shoulder. Perform twenty repetitions.

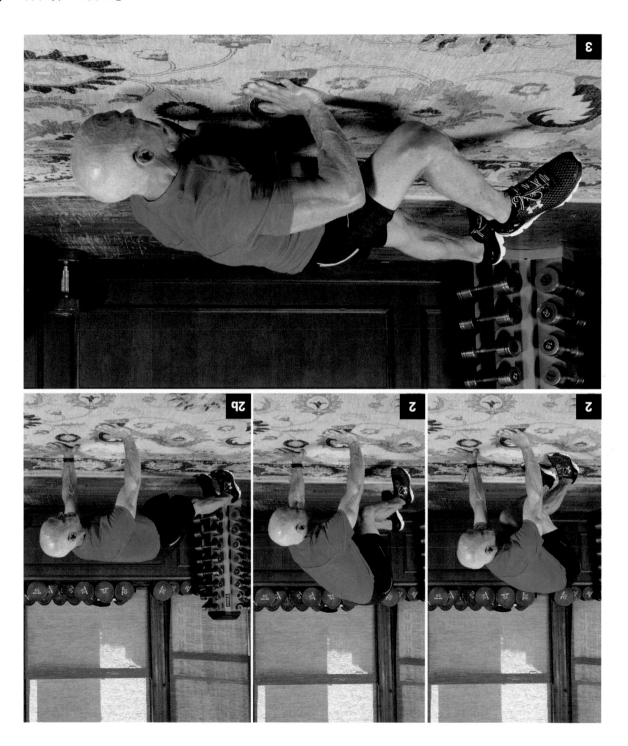

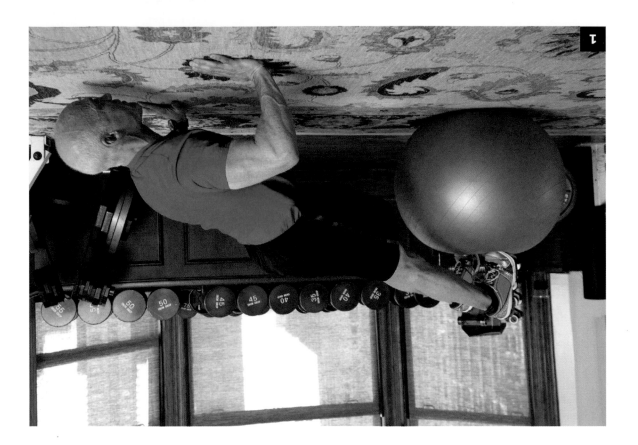

1.

Stability Ball Pike with a Knee Tuck

This exercise not only engages the core, but also strengthens the arms and lower back.

1 Walk into a pushup position with the balls of your feet on the stability ball and your palms on the floor under your chest. Keep your abs tight and don't allow your hips to sag downward.

2 Lift your hips up into a pike position and return to the starting position.

3 Keeping your hips aligned, bring your knees to your chest and return to the starting position. That's one rep; complete fifteen.

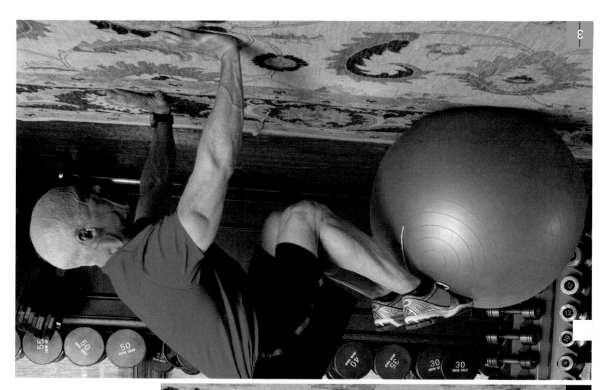

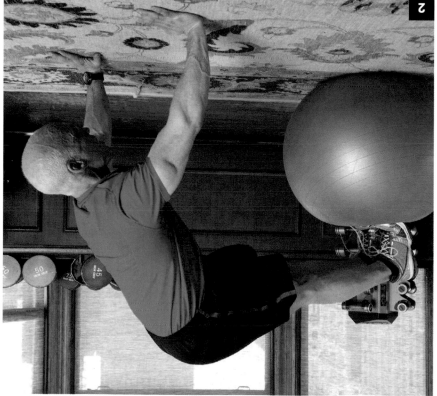

Plié Toe Squats with Lateral Raises

Work your butt, inner thighs, abs, and shoulders all at the same time. It's very economical!

1 Start with a wide-stance squat and hold a pair of dumbbells (or water bottles) at your sides.

2 Simultaneously raise your heels and squat—your thighs should be parallel to the floor—and lift your arms out to the side. Do fifteen repetitions.

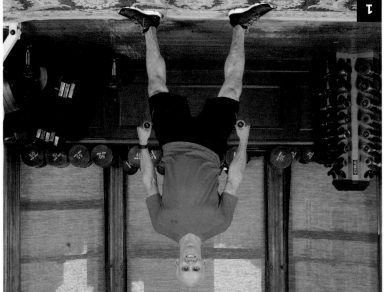

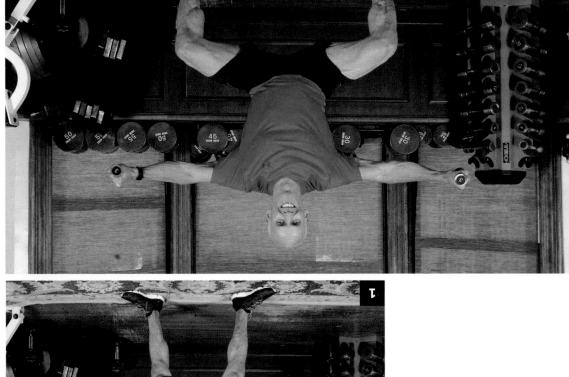

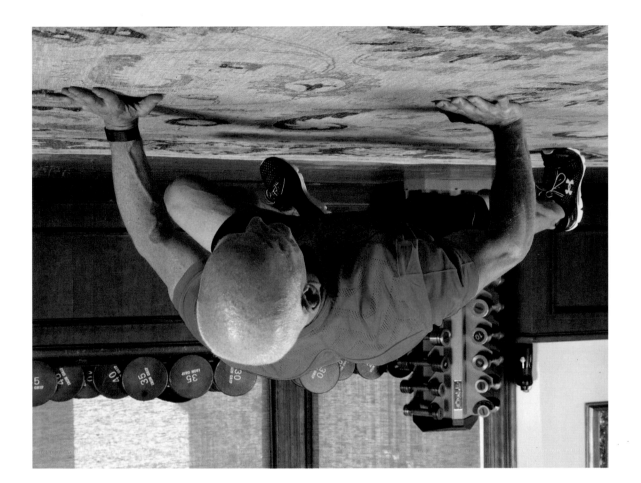

Spiderman Crawls

Are you ready to engage your inner Spidey?

1 Kneel on all fours with your knees under your hips and your hands under your chest. Extend your right arm and left leg.

2 Crawl forward, as Spiderman would crawl up a wall, extending your opposite limbs. Each time you crawl forward, lower yourself into an off-center pushup. For example, if your right arm and left leg are extended, bend both elbows and lower your chest to the floor. Complete twenty repetitions.

EXPRESS FULL-BODY PLANK WORKOUT

For those times when you want a change of pace, try my full-body plank workout. The following are some of the plank variations I've tried myself and with my clients. You will complete fifteen repetitions for each exercise. This workout, a full-body workout, can be used as a five-minute circuit workout for all three body types.

Plank with Knee Tuck to Hip Abduction

1 Start in a plank position (1a). Bring your right knee in toward your left shoulder (1b), then extend your leg back and out to the side (i.e., hip abduction) (1c). That's one repetition.

2 Repeat fifteen times with each leg.

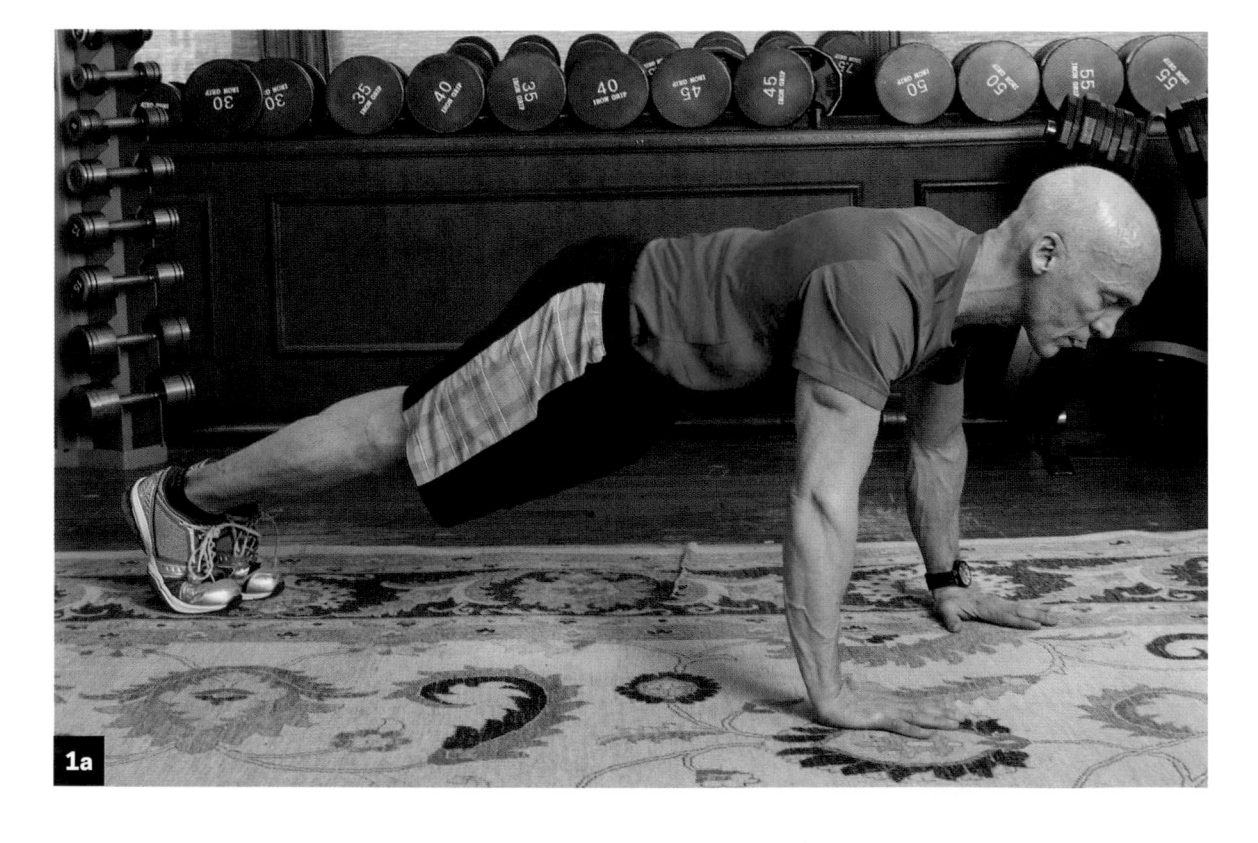

1a

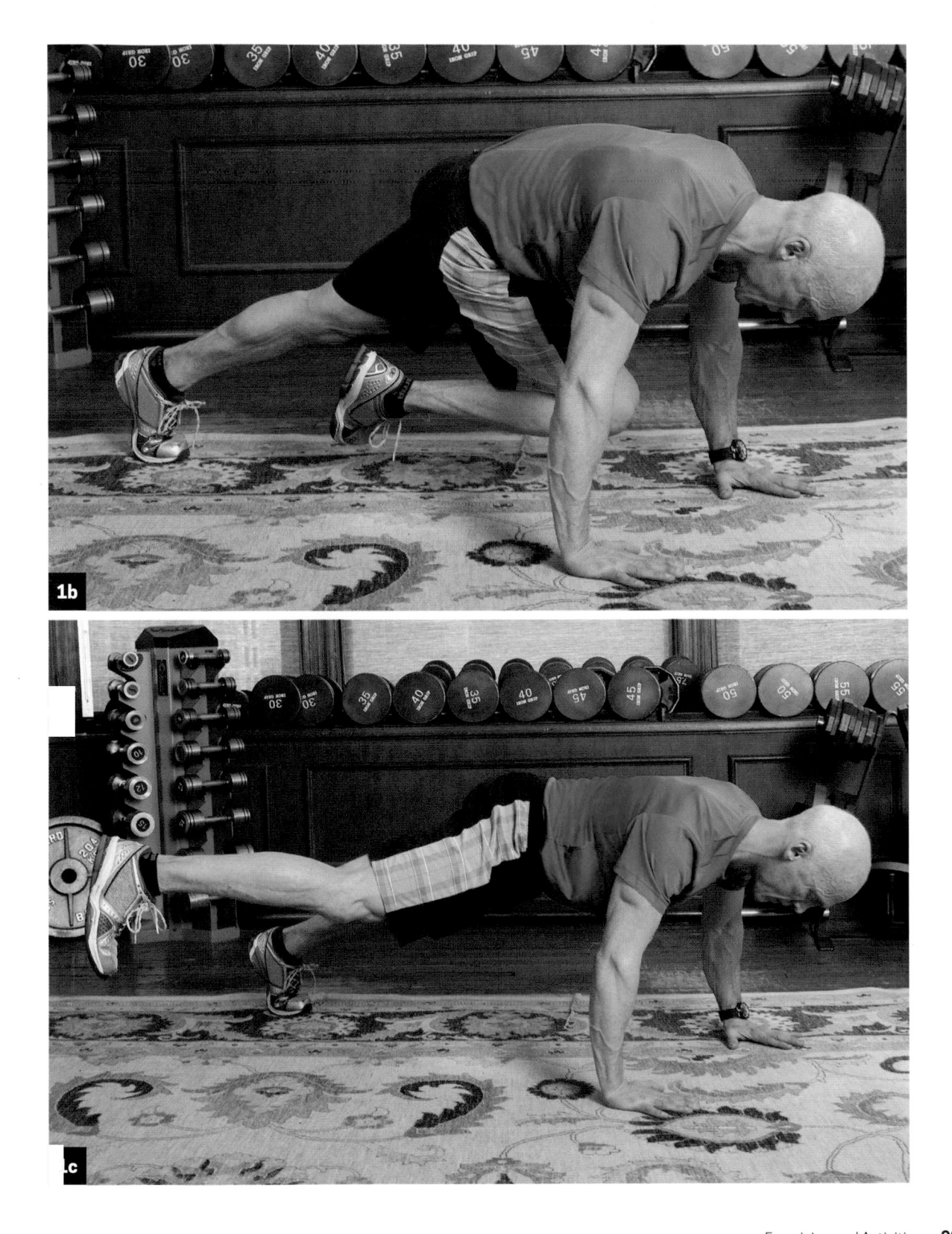

1b

1c

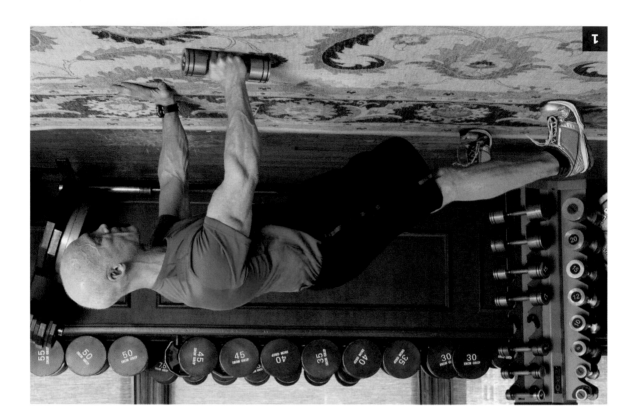

Plank with Dumbbell Row to Triceps Extension

1 Start in a plank position with a dumbbell (or water bottle) in your hand.

2 Pull up your right arm (2a), keeping it close to your side, and immediately extend your arm back to engage your triceps (2b). Repeat fifteen times on each side.

Kate Upton, in particular, is one of my clients that uses this workout when she's travelling.

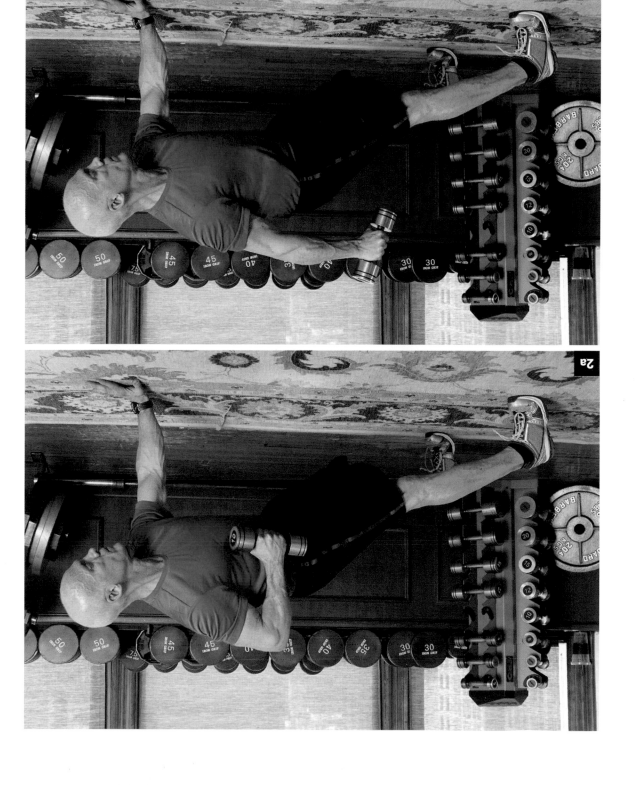

Plank with Front Raise to Side Lateral

1 Start in a plank position with a dumbbell (or a water bottle) in your hand.

2 Raise your right arm out to the side and parallel to the floor (2a), and then forward in front of your body (2b).

3 Repeat fifteen times on each side.

This workout is no joke! You can do it!

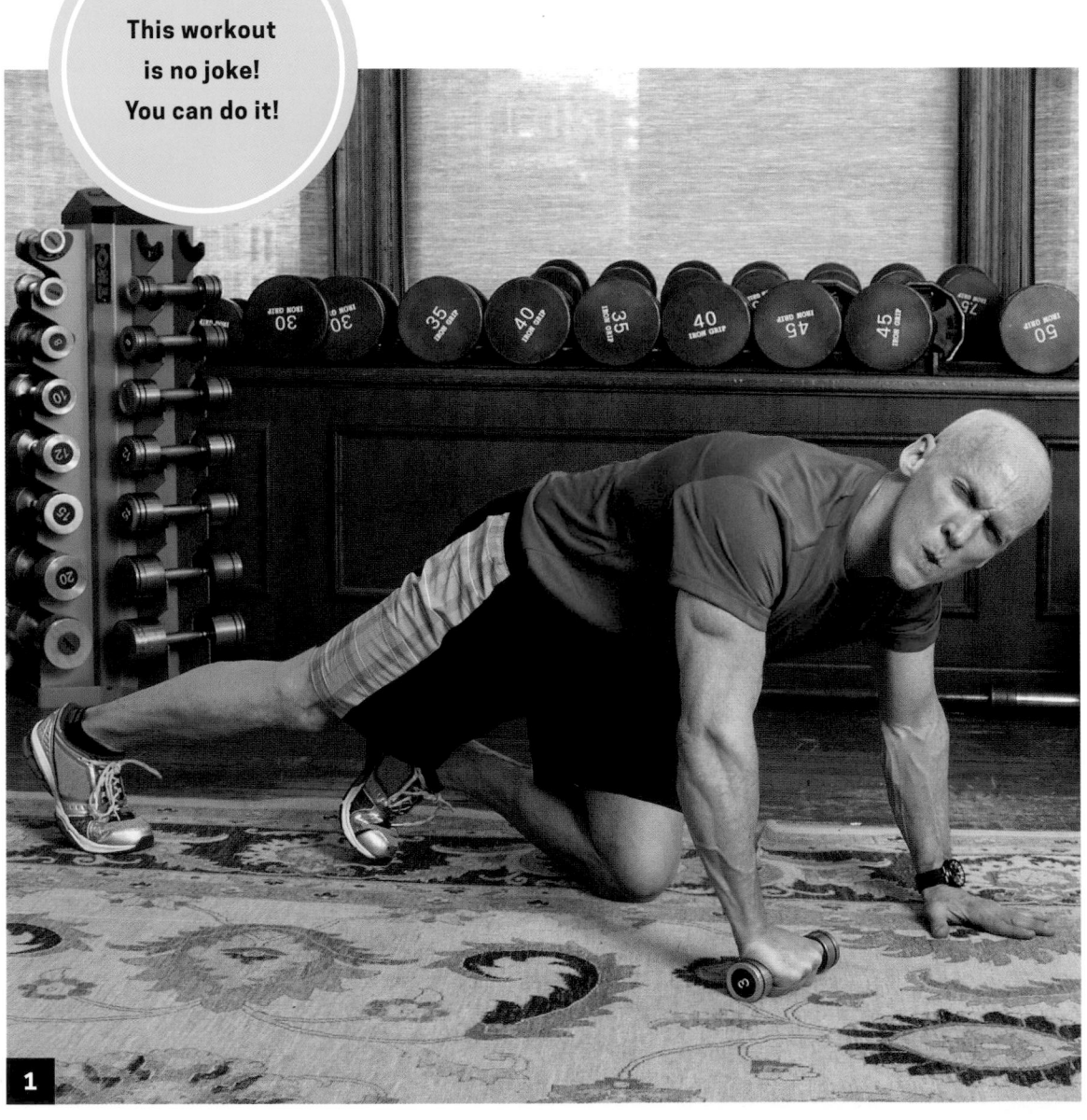

1

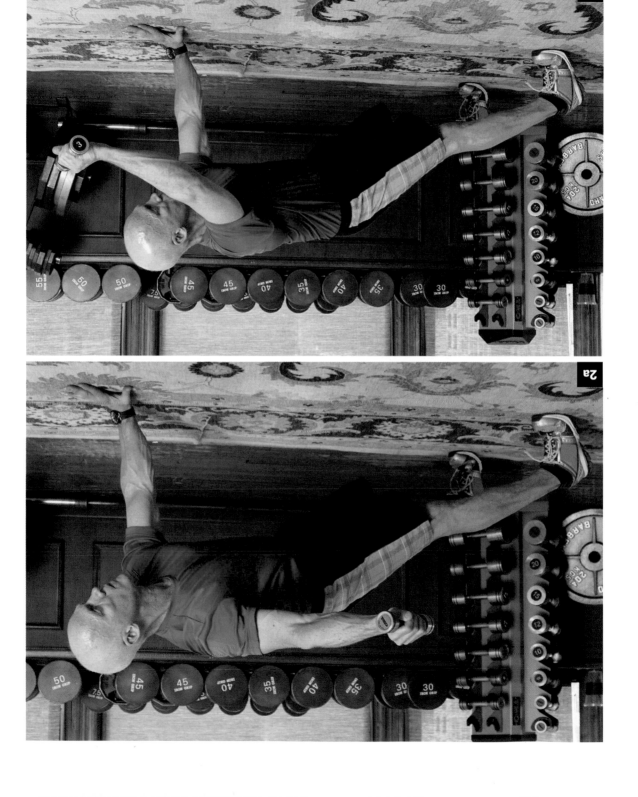

Side Plank Oblique Crunches
(see photos page 69)

1 Position yourself in a side plank, resting on your right forearm with your left arm behind your head.

2 Bring your left elbow in toward your belly and then return to the starting position. Do fifteen repetitions on each side.

Plank with Shoulder Taps

1 Start in a plank position.

2 Alternate tapping your hands to the opposite shoulder. Focus on keeping your core engaged and hips aligned, not wiggling.

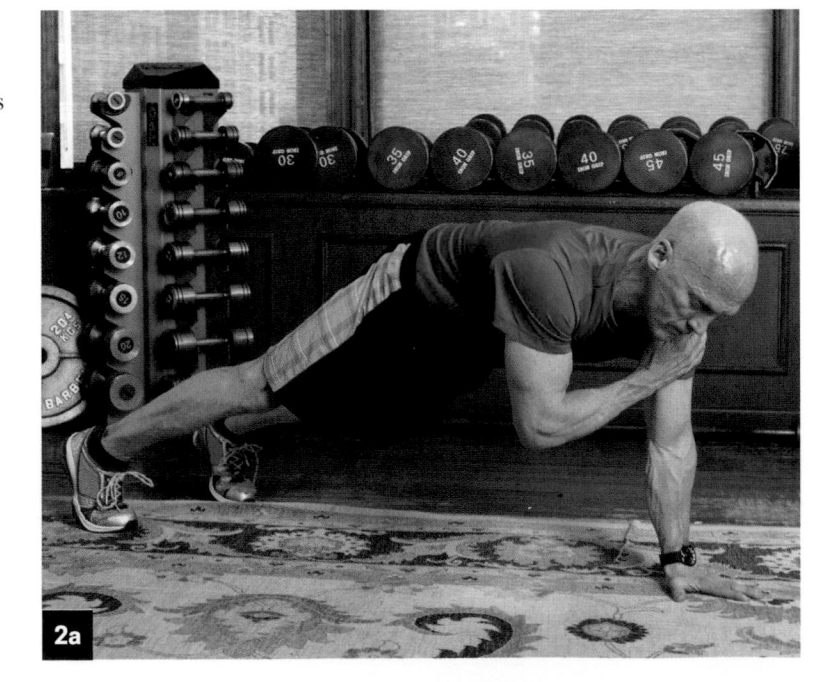

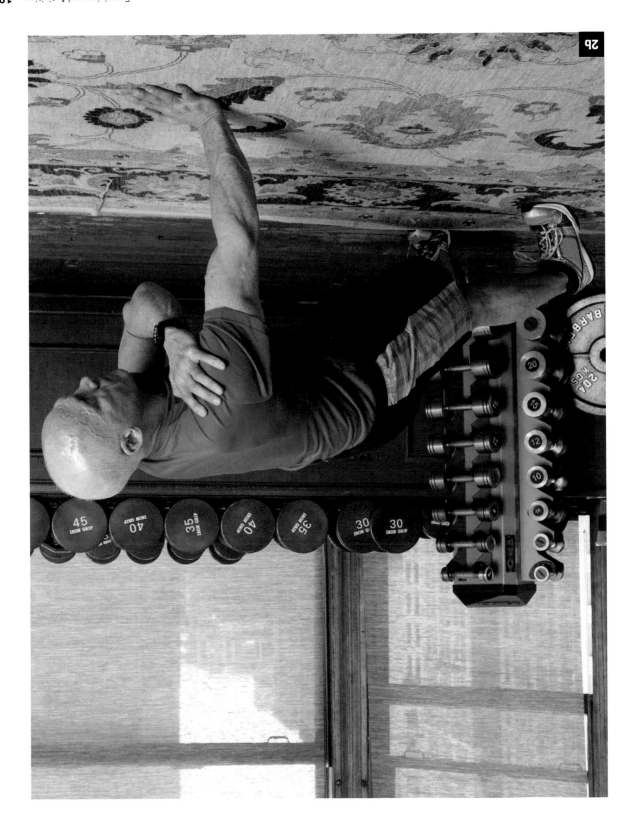

2b

FIVE-MINUTE CARDIO CIRCUITS

This five-minute cardio workout is great for days when you really want to get your blood pumping. It's not a routine for the five-day plan, but it is great for maintenance.

1 **Rowing machine:** Do 250-meter sprints with thirty seconds rest in between each sprint. Work up to three sprints.

2 **Treadmill:** Do thirty-second sprints that push you past your comfort zone. Repeat three times.

3 **Jump rope:** Perform one minute of high-intensity jumping and then do a thirty-second plank. Repeat three times.

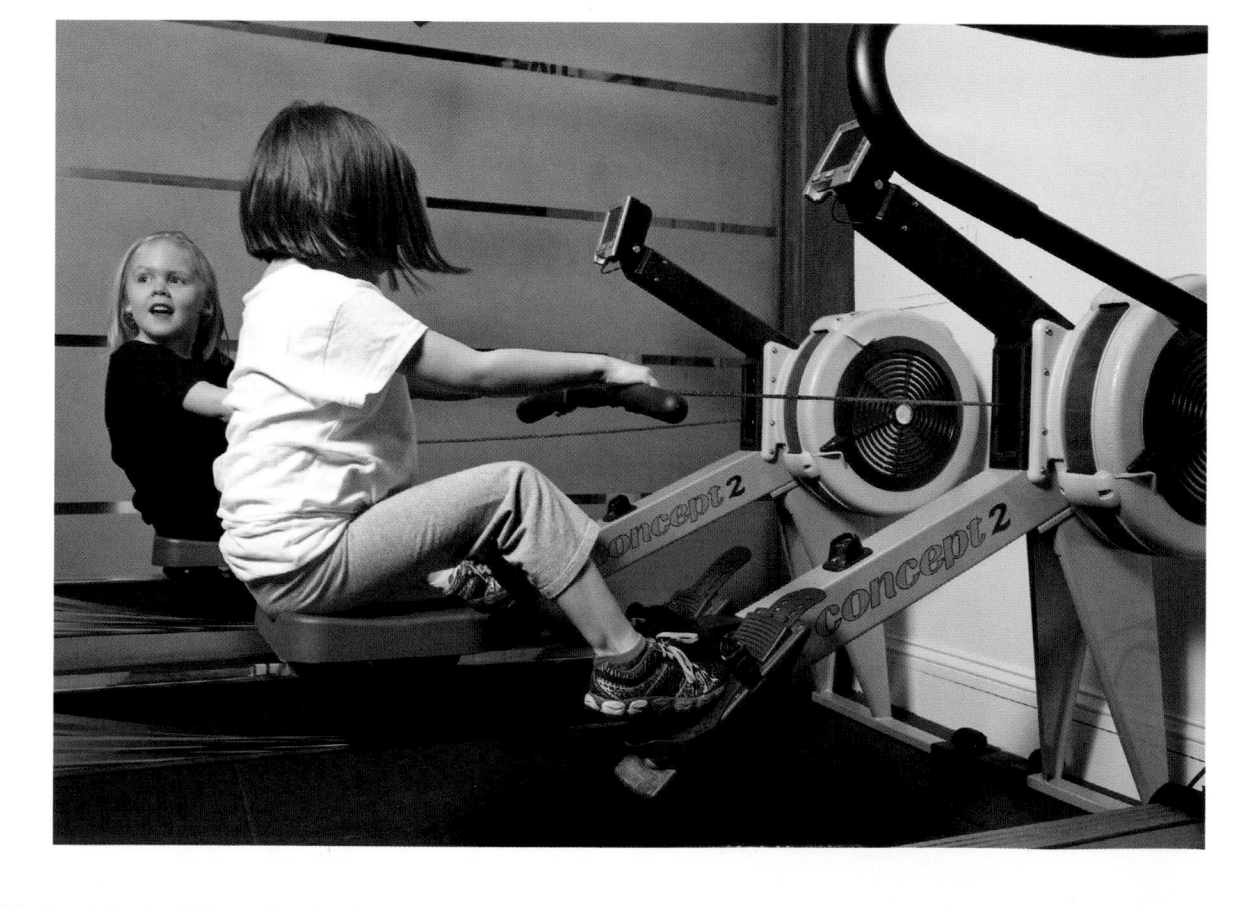

Making Cardio Work

Even though the 5-5-5 Program uses the power of HIIT, you may enjoy doing longer cardio routines when you're in the maintenance mode part of the program. Longer workouts can give you some needed personal time or let you burn off steam. To make the most out of any cardio routine, do the following:

Connect your mind and body. The concept of mind-body training is as important when doing cardio. No mindless workouts. They're a total waste of time.

- Disconnect from phones, tablets, and television. Whether doing your five-minute circuit or forty-five minutes on the treadmill or elliptical machine, visualize the calories burning, body fat melting, and muscles toning for maximum effect.

- Change it up. Doing the same "forty-five minutes on the elliptical" is neither productive nor interesting. Our bodies are very clever and need to be tricked by mixing up the routine a little. One cardio prescription that has worked well for my clients is starting with 2,500 meters on the rowing machine, which should take you between ten and twelve minutes. Follow this with a one-mile (1.6 km) sprint on the treadmill at between 7.5 and 8.0 mph (12 to 13 kmh) (or higher if you are able to). Finish with thirty minutes on the elliptical machine. My new favorite is the Octane lateral, which really blasts your thighs and glutes.

- Focus on duration first, intensity second. I'm often asked the question about whether duration or intensity is more important. One of the common mistakes people make when starting a cardio program is going hard and short. Instead, build up stamina and muscle strength first and then up the intensity.

- Don't lose heart. Look, I'll be the first to tell you that extended periods of time spent in the cardio room can be as stimulating as watching paint dry. But the reality is, there's no getting around it. Young or old, cardiovascular health is vitally important to overall wellness.

I have also included tips for maximizing the effects of the most common types of cardiovascular exercise:

Treadmill: If you are unable (or unwilling) to run, try walking on the treadmill at an incline. Warm up at 3.0 mph (4.8 kmh) and 2 percent incline and after a minute, up the speed (if you feel comfortable to) to 3.5 mph (5.6 kmh) and 5 percent incline. You will soon build up confidence, stamina, and energy to take it up to 10 percent and beyond (get ready for a major glutes burn) and vary the speed between 3.5 and 4.0 mph (5.6 to 6.4 kmh).

Elliptical machine: Most elliptical machines allow you to vary both stride length—the larger the number, the closer you are to simulating running—and incline to blast your quads, hip flexors, glutes, and hamstrings. Challenge yourself. I also recommend alternating going forward and reverse every few minutes. My new favorites—the Octane Lateral—really blasts you outer thighs and glutes; and the Octane Runner (with increasing stride) simulates running without the impact.

Gauntlet (stair climber): I don't think any cardio machine elicits more cries of protestation than this one. Here, a little bit goes a long way to delivering an effective sweat and fat burn. Ten to fifteen minutes at level 10, doing a crossover step, facing right, then left on the machine is as challenging and effective as thirty minutes on the elliptical machine.

Rowing machine: This is still my favorite go-to cardio machine for full-body conditioning. Start at 500-meter intervals, making sure your core is engaged, and press with your legs as you snap with your arms for maximum results. Once you have the form down, increase in 500-meter increments weekly or biweekly.

Versa climber: This machine is not for the faint of heart. For maximum effect and staying power, keep your core engaged and stick out your butt as you climb to exotic places like the Washington Monument and the Eiffel Tower.

FAMILY MOVEMENT, FAMILY FUN

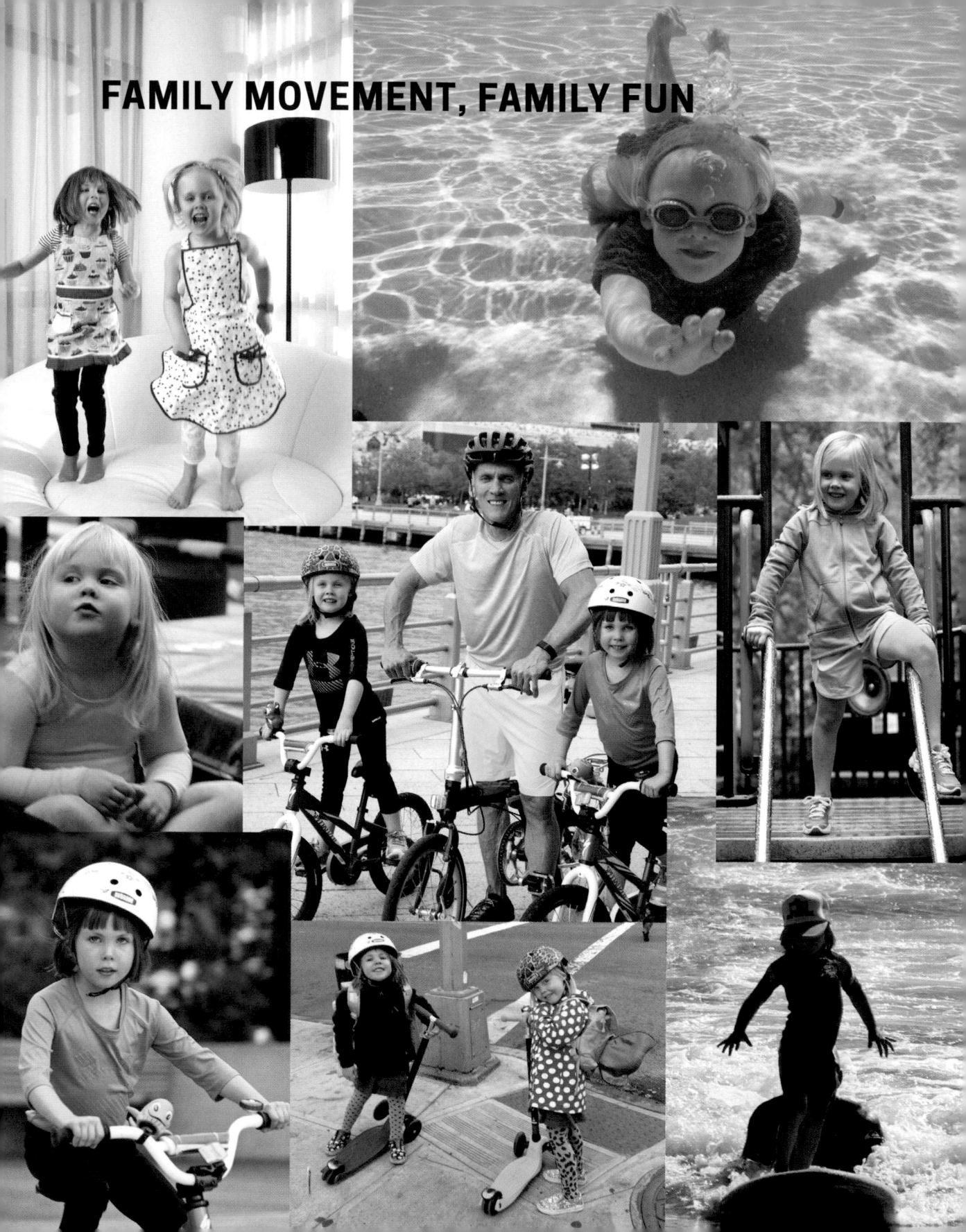

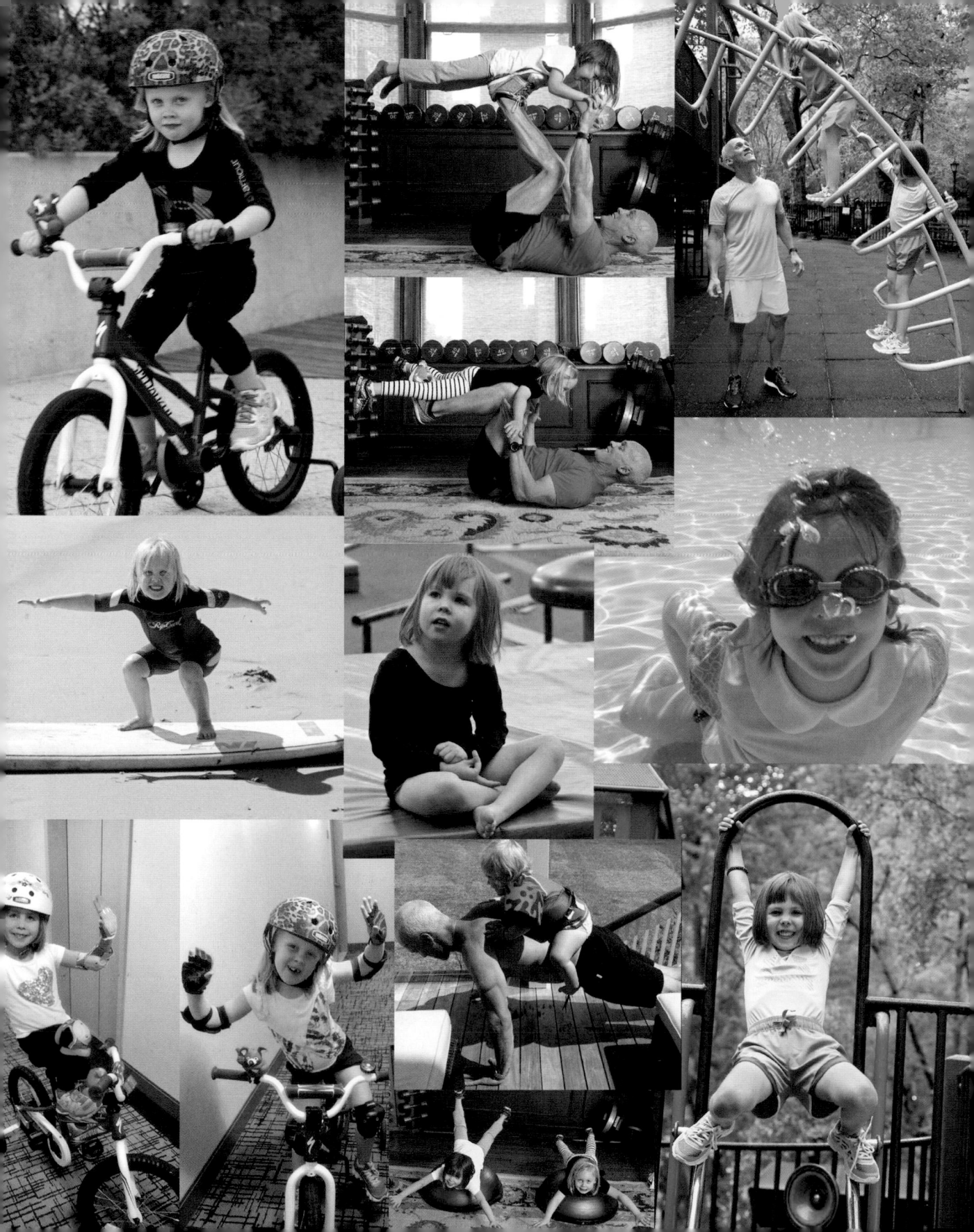

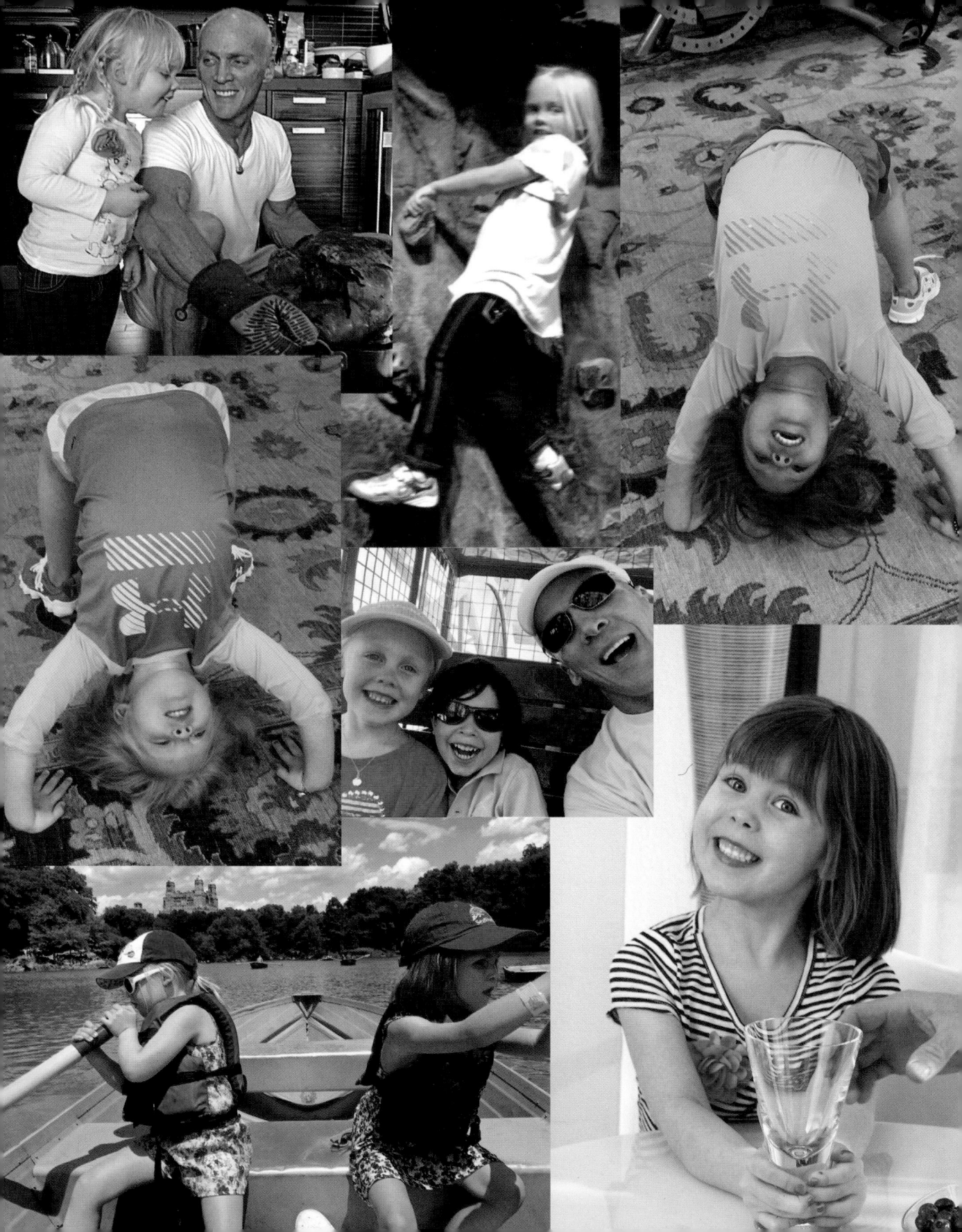

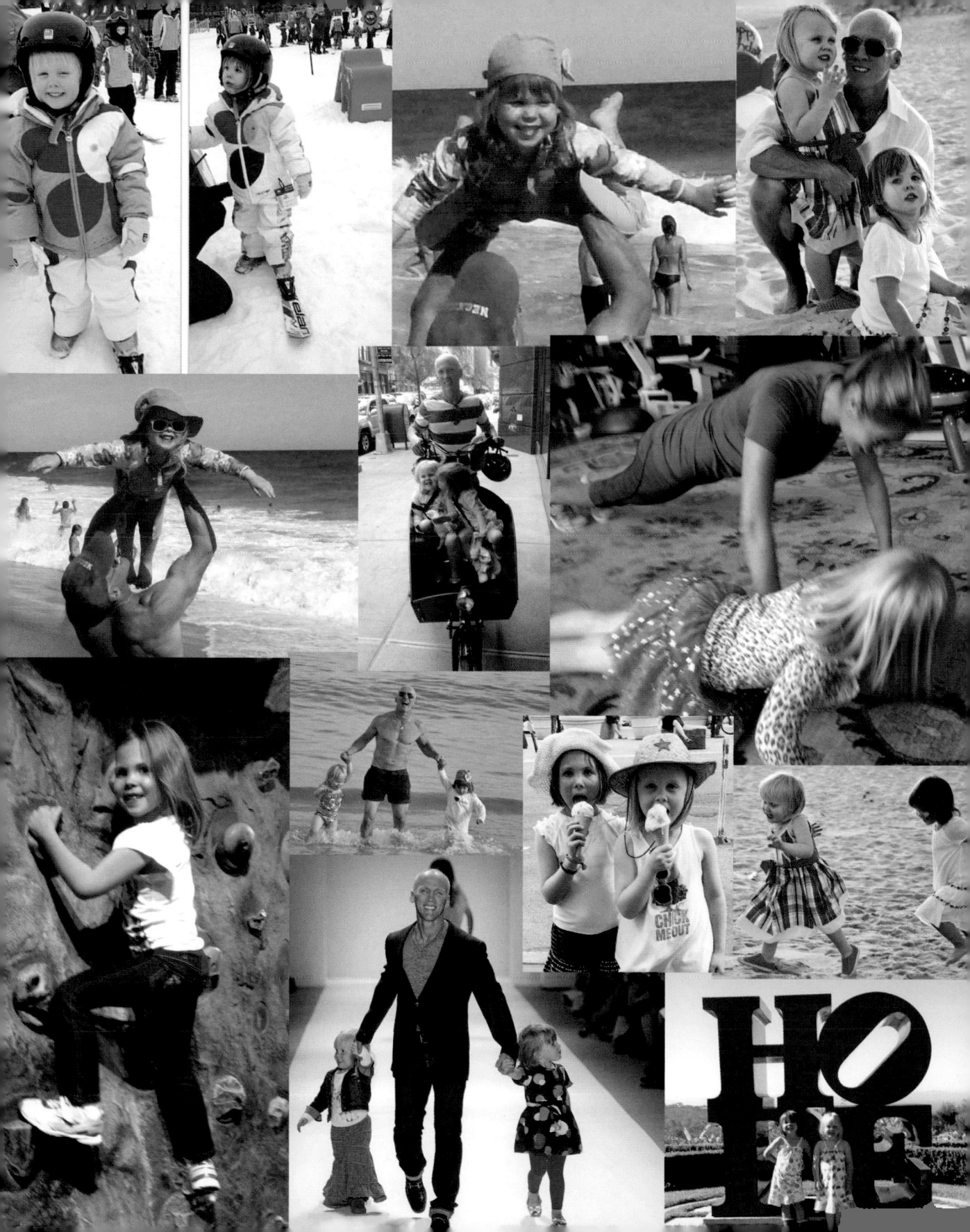

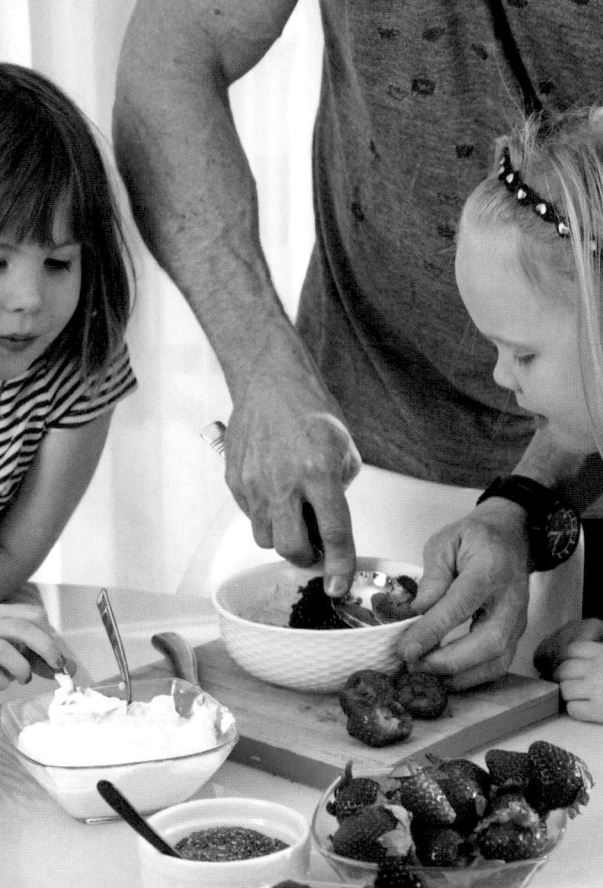
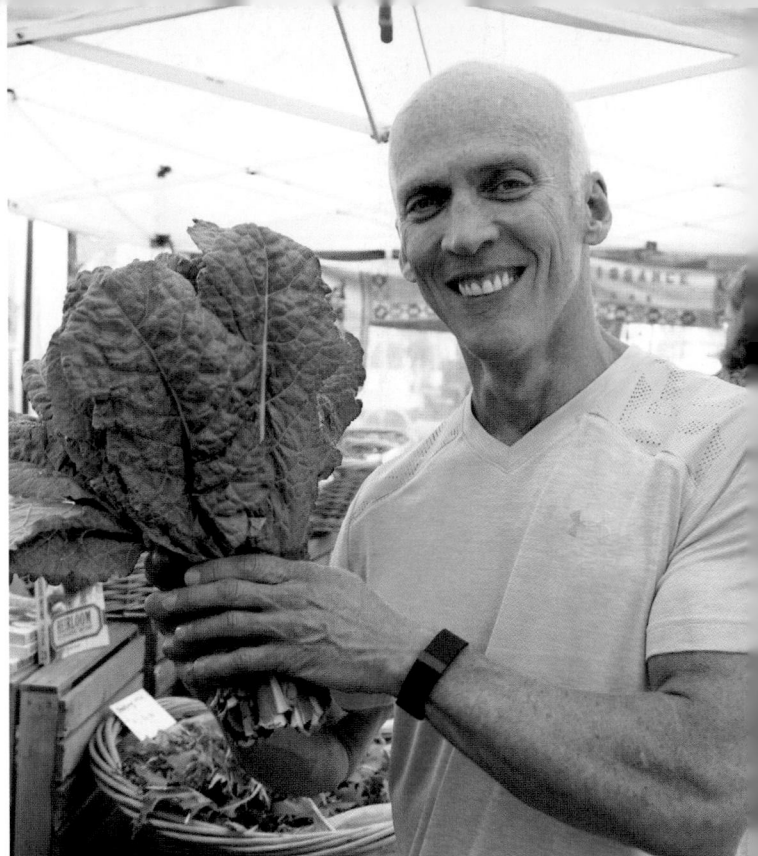

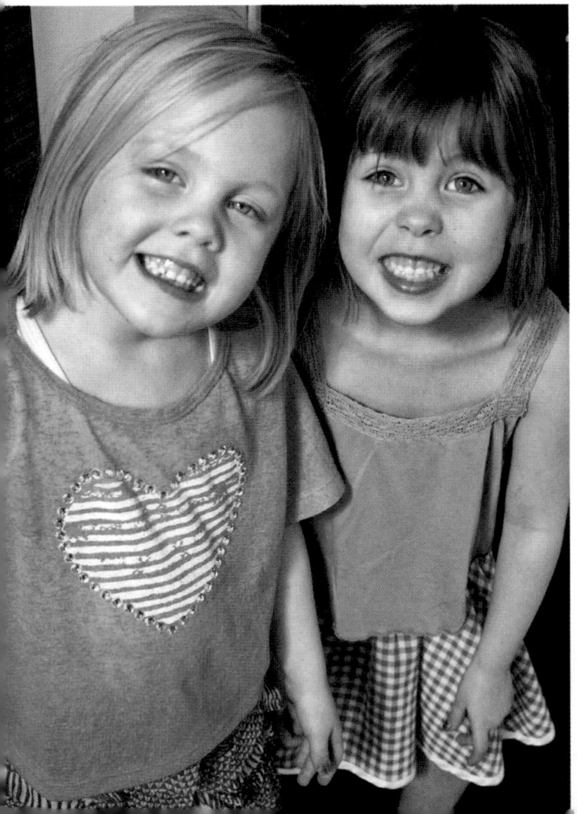

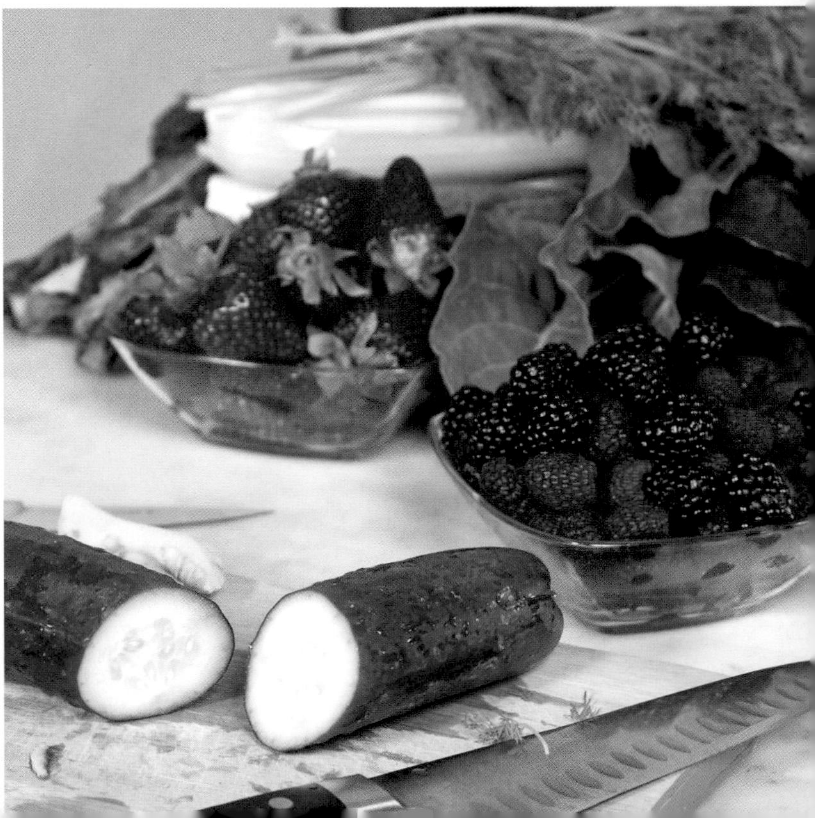

Chapter 3

NUTRITION, FOOD, AND FAMILY

WHY ARE FAMILY FOOD RITUALS IMPORTANT?

A baby cries and a mother and father don't know what to do. Our immediate response is give the baby a bottle, he or she must be hungry. We are conditioned from an early age to believe that food will be the answer—at times celebratory, consolatory, and always life-sustaining. Looking back on my own childhood, I remember with great fondness the emphasis placed on sitting down as a family to enjoy a home-cooked meal. It was at the kitchen table where all the important discussions took place—events of the day that happened at school, work, and home. My grandmother lived with us from the time I was five until I went to college, and the kitchen was her domain. She scheduled, planned, shopped, and cooked the majority of the meals, the exception being two of mom's special dishes: spaghetti and meatballs and frank-and-bean casserole. Grandma cooked with a full heart and took great pride in watching us clean our plates.

When I became a parent myself at age forty-eight, my life was turned upside down. My rituals pre-babies—work, workouts, how/what/when I ate, and personal time—changed dramatically, all in the most gloriously rewarding way. I will always cherish our first family ritual, cradling both Emilia and Francesca in my arms and curling up on my brown leather recliner to feed them their bedtime bottles. Inevitably, the three of us fell asleep cuddling, a sated and content family. By the time the girls were two, they were picking me up at my fitness club for our daily lunch. For two hours, I didn't think about work, emails, or clients. We shared laughs, hugs, and food. Carving out time from my hectic workday to lunch with my girls fed and nourished our hearts, souls, and bellies. Oh how I miss that family food ritual. Lunch has never been the same!

Fast forward to the present. My twins are five years old. As the head of the house, I know that how we treat food in the home will teach my children how to eat, and establishing a healthy approach to nutrition—both inside and out of the home—is one of the most important lessons I can share with them.

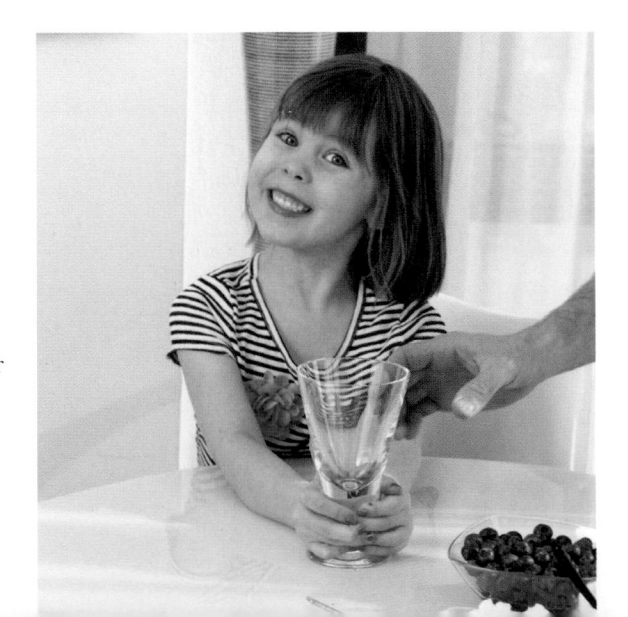

Food plays a vital role in our family life, and I have embraced and expanded the rituals I grew up with, making them much more democratic and inclusive. Eating home-cooked meals together as a family is something that, despite my busy schedule, I am reluctant to miss. In many respects, the kitchen is the heart and soul of my house; it's one of the places we nourish our minds, bodies, and souls.

Unlike my role in my own childhood, Emilia and Francesca weigh in with suggestions about what we should buy and prepare for meals. One of our favorite Saturday rituals is going to the Union Square Farmers Market, and fall wouldn't be complete without a trip to a local orchard to pick fresh apples, pears, and pumpkins. On our weekly jaunts to Whole Foods, each girl selects one item she would like included in our meals. They have learned to look and often ask for organic fruits, vegetables, and dairy. There is of course the "discussion" about whether they need a bagel to nibble on at the grocery store, and in that moment, grabbing a whole-wheat bagel seems the lesser of evils.

You naturally pass on to your children lessons about the way you eat and the amount of exercise and movement you embrace. I never sat my girls down for a nutrition class or to explain the importance of movement, but these have become a natural part of the fabric of their lives simply because they watch me. Family food rituals are also important for their ability to help establish a healthy, balanced relationship with food and eating. So whether it's grocery shopping with your family, planning and preparing healthful meals at home, or choosing the time and type of occasional treat, regular family meals offer invaluable bonding and often, teaching moments.

As the girls have gotten older, they have shown increasing interest in helping me plan and prepare meals. Whether cracking and mixing eggs for french toast or mixing the ground turkey breast for turkey burgers, they have become active participants in the kitchen. We have created another family food ritual.

I'm sure as you read this, you are thinking of your own family food rituals because we all have them. I cherish my rituals with Emilia and Francesca and look forward to sharing many more in the years to come.

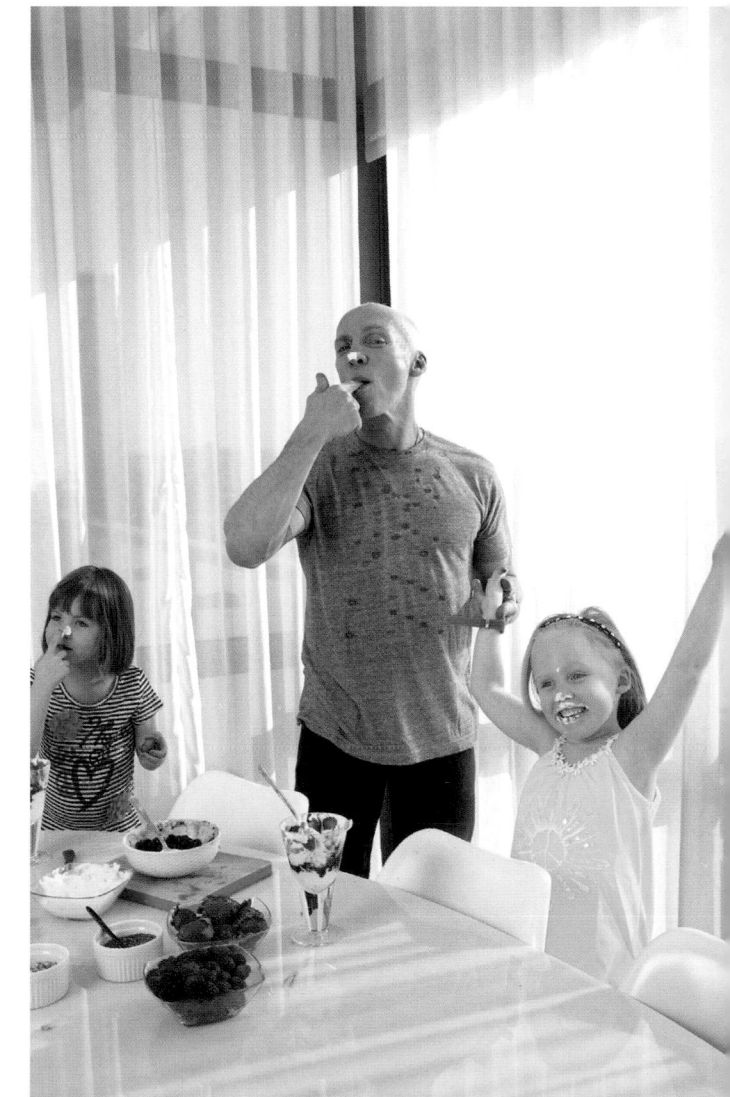

FIVE RULES FOR OPTIMAL NUTRITION

No fitness and wellness program would be successful without the support of and adherence to a solid nutrition plan. I will now set forth the Five Rules for Optimal Nutrition. You will need to stick to these rules strictly for the five-day portion of the plan. (Meal plans for this part of the program can be found in chapter 5 on page 206.)

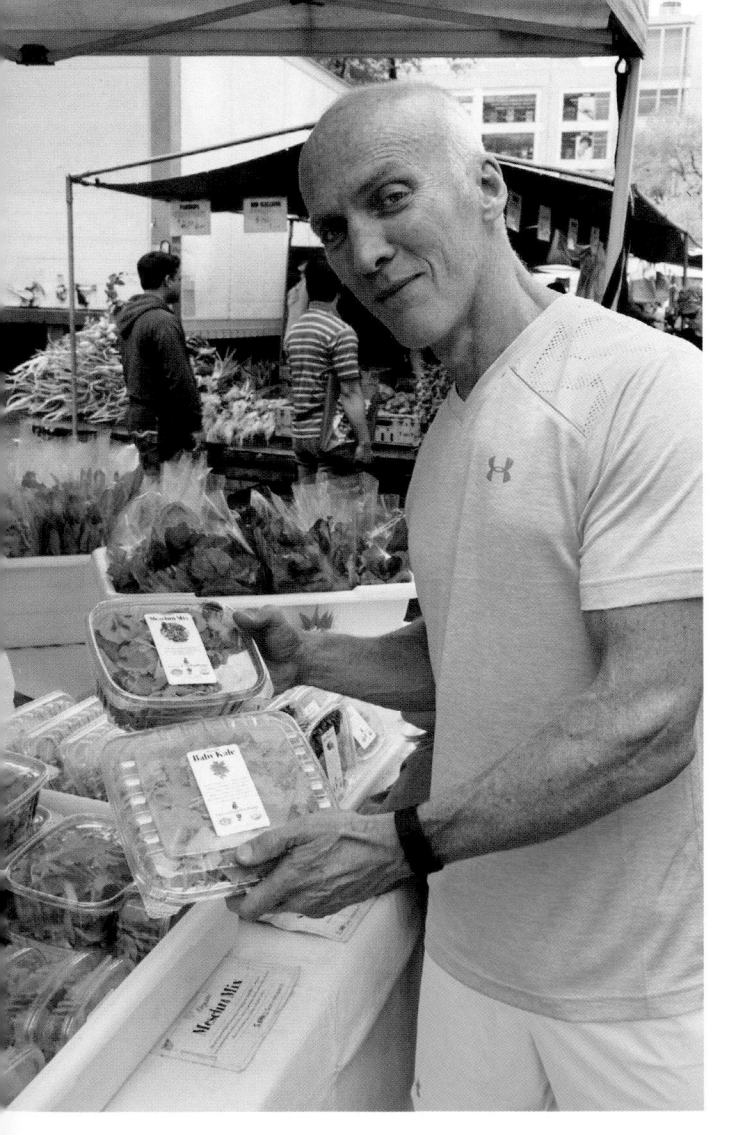

This book lays out two simultaneous notions. There's the 5-5-5 Program: five days, five exercises, five pounds. This contains the overriding principles of exercise and good, balanced eating that will apply to you and your family after the initial five days. The 5-5-5 Program is your quick-start weight-loss program, and that extends into your Ultimate Family Wellness Plan.

After those initial five days, the rules will still apply, but you'll add in more kid-friendly foods found in the "ABC" section of this chapter. By following these rules and those ABCs, you'll have a greater understanding of how these foods—good and not so good—affect your daily life, overall energy, productivity, mood, and emotions. With this knowledge, you'll be able to choose the right foods in the right proportions for the right times (and I make it especially easy with the kid-tested recipes in chapter 4). You'll be stronger and more energized than ever. And if you cheat now and again, don't feel like you failed and have to give up. Life happens. Do the best you can, and you'll be amazed by how good you feel.

RULE 1: No alcohol.

This includes wine, Champagne, beer, and hard alcohol. These are absolute no-nos during the five days of the program. Full disclosure, I often lead my clients by example, but I just returned from a tasty Italian meal at my good friend Danny Meyer's restaurant Marta where I enjoyed a couple glasses of Barolo. After all, red wine is heart-healthy (I tell myself) and my father swears by the "potassium" he derived from the Champagne he drank post-marathons. Even though a *very* occasional glass or two can be a treat (and often the go-to at the end of a long, stressful day), once you've achieved your fitness goals and are in maintenance mode, there is almost no nutritional benefit to the calories consumed by drinking alcohol. You might be asking, what harm can a glass or two do every night? The answer is plenty.

Your liver recognizes the byproducts of alcohol as toxins, so your body stops processing nutrients from the food you've eaten while it takes care of the toxins first. As a result, your body burns empty alcohol calories (i.e., those low in nutrients) for energy instead of burning fat and carbs, all while leaving behind the digestion of nutrient-rich food.

Alcohol also breaks down amino acids and stores them as fat. When you consume more calories than you burn—a likely scenario when alcohol is part of your meal—your body stores the excess as fat. By the time your body gets around to burning food calories, it may not need the energy and could end up storing the extra calories you've eaten as fat cells. In conclusion, I think the possible health benefits (e.g., heart health with red wine) of drinking alcohol don't outweigh the risks.

As a practical aside, during the five days on the program, there is no room for hangovers or post-drink sluggishness. You need to be fresh, focused, and on top of your game to achieve the desired results.

RULE 2: No highly processed or refined foods.

Don't get me wrong. I'm not saying carbohydrates are bad, but rather it's the highly processed, refined carbohydrates stripped of nutrients and dietary fiber, leaving you with just simple sugars, that I'm against. The difference between whole-wheat and refined flour—such as in whole-wheat pasta and "regular" pasta—is this nutrient-stripping, refining process, and it's those refined foods you need to avoid. The following are two of my favorite, nutrient-rich, go-to whole foods: quinoa and brown rice. The rules of the five-day program require you to stick to greens and protein, however, so you will abstain from eating them until after the program.

As a parent, I make healthy choices when food shopping for Emilia and Francesca, but it is easy to be misled. We are surrounded by the omnipresent fast-food offerings on every street in New York City, and practically every aisle in the grocery store overflows with packaged foods. It's easy to fall for the seemingly healthy boxes of organic refined carbs: gluten-free crackers, low-fat cookies, "barely" there wheat bread with corn syrup. They seem like good choices, but they are, in fact, packed with refined carbohydrates.

Refined carbs digest quickly, which can lead to surges in blood-sugar levels. Moments after consuming them, you'll be hungry and craving more. These carbohydrates not only fail to give your body the right nutrition, but they also cause you to gain weight through overeating. To top it off, most refined carbs are often loaded with sodium, and many are high in unhealthy saturated fat.

For this program—and optimal health as well—it's best to avoid refined carbs as much as possible. You get little nutrition from them, and you may find that after a blood-sugar surge, your energy drops. They give you an instant energy burst, nothing more, and that's the last thing you need while on the 5-5-5 Program.

Throughout this program (and hopefully beyond), you will stick with whole foods such a vegetables and eggs as much as possible. Whole foods taste good and offer optimal fuel, energy, and longevity. (You'll see a great recipe in chapter 4 where I use kamut or brown rice pasta instead of regular pasta.) Even when I serve Emilia and Francesca pasta, I always add some extra nutritional value by topping it with a fresh tomato sauce (full of nutrients such as vitamin C and lycopene, among others) and using healthy fats such as olive oil to slow the absorption of the processed carb (i.e., pasta). Remember, food is fuel and as such, meant to optimally fuel you. If the food you consume makes you feel sluggish and lethargic, you are not eating the right foods.

RULE 3: No added sugars or artificial sweeteners.

They might make foods taste better, but added sugars such as sucrose and high-fructose corn syrup equal unnecessary calories. They contain a whole bunch of calories with no proteins, essential fats, or nutrients and are therefore referred to as "empty" calories.

There are no proteins, essential fats, vitamins, or minerals in sugar . . . just pure energy. There is often a direct correlation between highly processed/refined foods and added sugars. Soda, for example, is the absolute worst—one twelve-ounce can (355 ml) contains nine teaspoons (36 g) of sugar. And according to recent studies, eating sugar increases your risk of dying from heart disease.

That said, fruit naturally contains sugar, and who doesn't love a refreshing bowl of organic berries. Although fruits have incredible health benefits, I need you to refrain from eating them during the five days on the program because of their sugar content.

As for artificial sweeteners, there isn't much good to say about them. In fact, research has shown they can cause myriad health problems. Avoid them from here on out. Here's a list of sweeteners to avoid during the five-day plan and ideally minimize from your pantry and diet after that:

- Table sugar
  (sucrose; may be cane sugar or beet sugar)

- Honey

- Agave

- Corn syrup

- Brown sugar

- Molasses

- Maple syrup

- Fructose (except that which naturally occurs in whole fruits, after you complete the plan)

- Maltose

- Dextrose (Any ingredient ending in "-ose" is a sugar, except for cellulose, which is plant fiber.)

- Splenda (mostly dextrose)

- Fruit juice concentrates

- Fruit juice (It's okay to use small amounts in recipes, and pure lemon and lime juices are fine.)

As a regular blogger for *The Huffington Post*, I often address family health concerns. In a post I wrote about my struggles with Halloween, I concluded that American children daily consume far too much added sugar. Excessive sugar can suppress the immune system, promote tooth decay, and cause weight gain and many weight-related issues. I believe foods that contain added sugars and artificial sweeteners should not be consumed during the 5-5-5 Program or, for that matter, ever. This goes for you and your family (with the exceptional, occasional gelato treat, of course).

RULE 4: Eat lean and clean proteins.

Proteins are essential for building and repairing cells and creating new muscle. I am often asked, what is the best source of protein? I'd like to shed some light on what I feel are the best. I am a big advocate of eating animals that swim and fly. Wild salmon, brook trout, turkey, chicken, and eggs are some of my favorite protein sources. If you are a vegetarian, choose from tofu, tempeh, and seitan. But regardless of whether your diet is Paleo, omnivore, herbivore, vegetarian, or vegan, you need protein.

When looking at the strongest sources of protein, I consider the foods with the highest protein-to-calorie ratio. Using that formula, here's what I come up with:

- Turkey or chicken breast (30 grams of protein, 1 gram of protein per 4.5 calories)

- Fish such as salmon, tuna, and halibut (26 grams of protein, 1 gram per 4.5 calories)

- Tofu (7 grams of protein, 1 gram per 7.4 calories)

- Beans (17 grams of protein, 1 gram per 10.4 calories)

- Eggs (13 grams of protein, 1 gram per 12 calories)

- Yogurt, milk, and soymilk (6 grams, 1 gram per 18 calories)

- Nuts and seeds such as pumpkin, almond, walnuts, pine nuts, and sesame seeds (33 grams of protein, 1 gram per 15.8 calories)

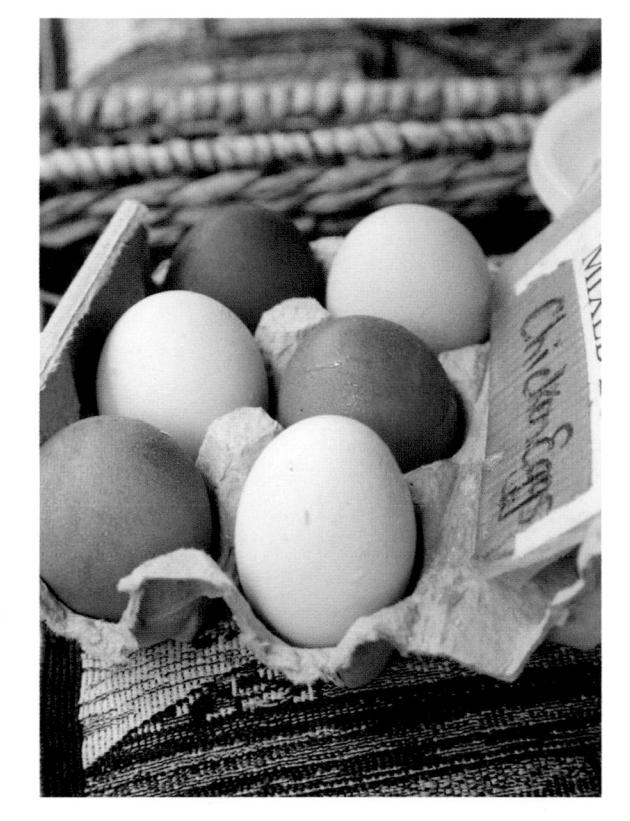

Make sure that your protein source is hormone-, pesticide-, and antibiotic-free. If available, choose organic lean meats and poultry. So much research has been done on the benefits of eating a "clean diet" free of pesticides, hormones, and chemicals. If you go to the trouble of choosing a lean chicken over a fatty steak, you should make sure the chicken is all it can be and nothing more. When it comes to seafood, my favorite is wild salmon. It is a highly nutritious food full of "good fats," but did you know that a four-ounce (115 g) serving of wild salmon also provides a full day's requirement of vitamin D? It is one of the few foods able to make that claim. That same piece of salmon also contains more than half the necessary vitamin B12, niacin, and selenium and is an excellent source of vitamin B6 and magnesium. Canned salmon also contains large amounts of calcium due to the fish bones.

RULE 5: Eat more fiber and dark leafy green vegetables.

"You got to eat your spinach baby . . . " (as Shirley Temple sang in one of her movies) and broccoli, kale, Brussels sprouts, and cauliflower to help keep your digestive tract moving, keep you regular, and prevent bloating. "Greens are the number one food you can eat regularly to help improve your health," says Jill Nussinow, M.S., R.D., a culinary educator in Northern California and the author of *The Veggie Queen*. That's because leafy vegetables are brimming with fiber, along with vitamins, minerals, and plant-based substances that may help protect you from heart disease, diabetes, and perhaps even cancer. Additionally, they are low in calories and a versatile delicious and nutritious part of your daily nutrition regimen. Emilia, Francesca, and I enjoy our greens raw in salads, roasted (especially Brussels sprouts, broccoli, and cauliflower), and as juice. I start every day with a green juice of kale, chard, cucumber, celery, fresh ginger, parsley, and dill.

Good Fats versus Bad Fats

You've probably heard that not all fats are created equal, but what does that mean? Well, saturated and trans fat are the bad guys, causing weight gain, clogging arteries, and offering little nutrition. They are found in fatty meat cuts, chicken skin, butter, whole-fat dairy, and many packaged and processed foods such as cookies, chips, fried foods, and candy.

The good guys are monounsaturated and polyunsaturated fats and omega-3s. These help your mental state stay balanced, keep you energized, and can even aid in controlling weight. You can find them in many natural oils such as olive, canola, and peanut oil, as well as in avocado, nuts, fatty fish, and tofu.

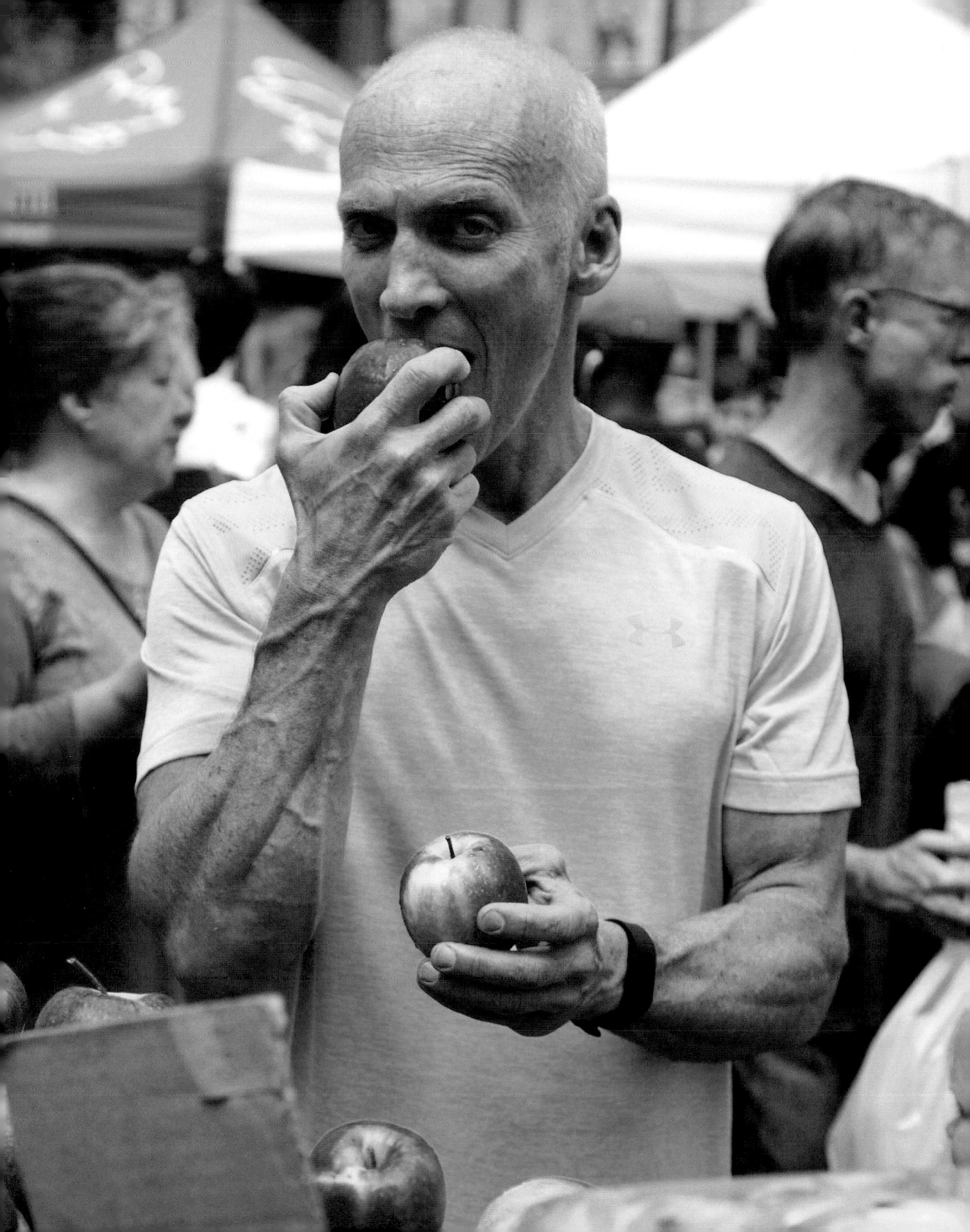

THE ABCs OF NUTRITION

In my international best-selling books, *The Ultimate New York Body Plan* and follow-up *The Ultimate New York Diet*, I promised the unthinkable: fourteen pounds (6.4 kg) in fourteen days and two dress sizes if you followed my training regimen and my ABC Rules of Nutrition. The rules were strict and the diet and calorie count restricted. I am very proud of the program and the life-transforming results realized by hundreds of thousands of people. The program is still available for those able to make the time commitment and of strong mind and body.

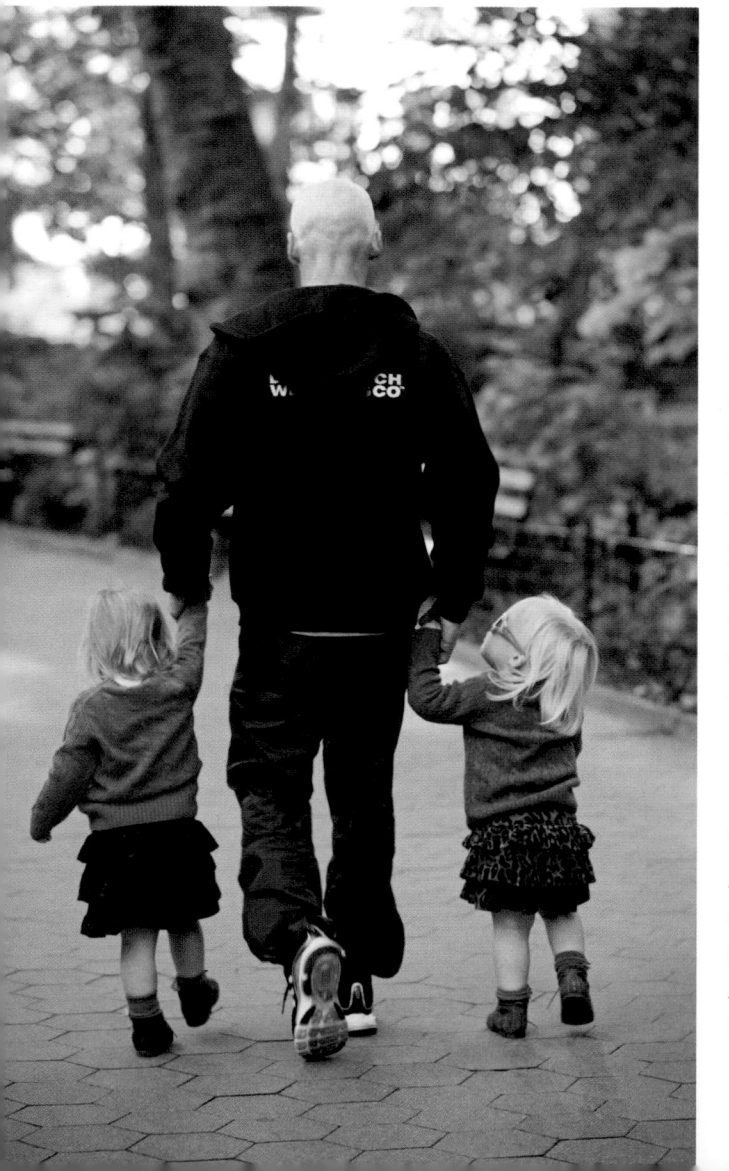

However, a lot has happened in my life since 2006. I have had great success but sadly, I have experienced great personal setbacks as well. My steadfast belief in God's greater purpose saw me through it all. I also think that as we get older, we evolve. After many years devoted to health and wellness and nurturing clients, family, and friends, I was ready for my next challenge: children. After all those years, I found what was really missing in my life. My guardian angels answered my prayers and with that, transformed my life forever. And with the birth of my twin girls, my inner child was reborn. I had the knowledge (and bruises) of decades of living life to the fullest with the promise of hope, possibility, and awe of a newborn child. Becoming a father at forty-eight years old was definitely challenging and a bit daunting, but the moment I cradled them in my arms, I knew that I was born to be a parent—I had realized my life-long dream.

ABCs Revisited

As my life has evolved and I have grown as a parent and as a person, I thought it was time to review, modify, and expand on my original concept of ABCs. The ABCs were created in 2004; it is now 2015 and so much has changed. As Emilia and

Francesca learned their ABCs, it was the perfect time for me to relearn mine. First, as a single father of twin girls, there are certain words that I have removed from my vocabulary. The word *fat* is never used to describe anything, and as Francesca was quick to point out to her kindergarten teacher, *diet* is a four-letter word that isn't in our lexicon. As I have relaxed—albeit, just a bit—with my approach to nutrition, I have also modified and expanded my ABC Rules of Nutrition.

The following is my broader and more inclusive list of the food groups and individual foods allowed on the Ultimate Family Wellness Plan, as well as the foods to limit and/or avoid. As with the Five Rules for Optimal Nutrition, you need to strictly adhere to the dos and don'ts of this list while on the five-day plan. In maintenance mode and beyond, the rules should be considered a blueprint and guide to help you toward an ultimate life of wellness. Built into the maintenance plan is an allowance for the occasional treat. Indulge sparingly and mindfully, and don't beat yourself up over it.

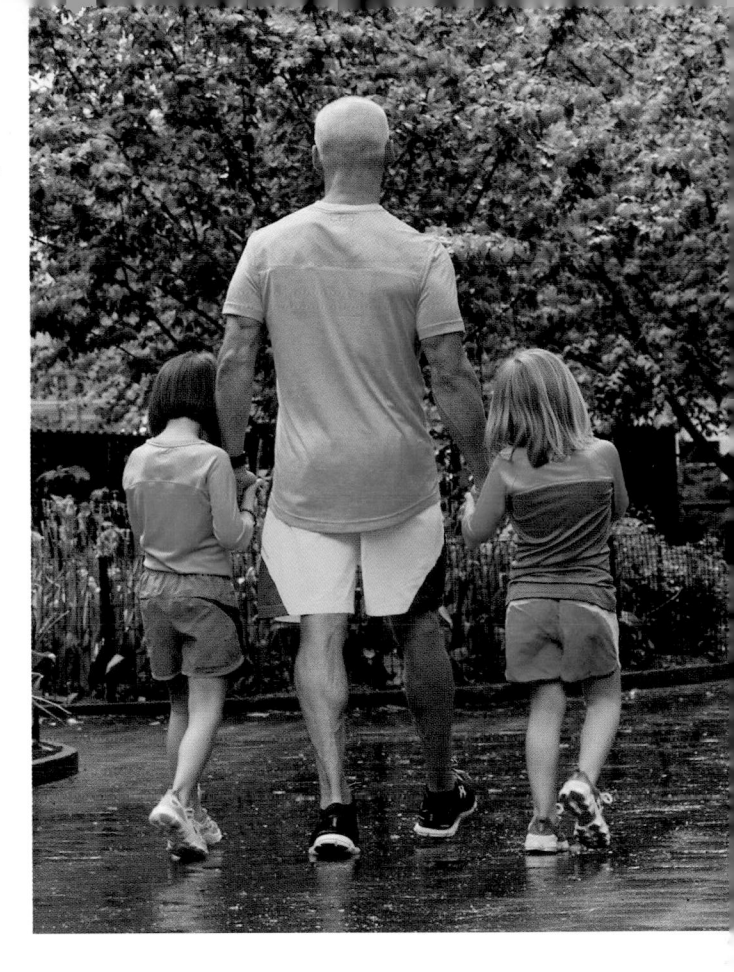

A

Alcohol is a total no-no. Once off of the program, a glass of wine, vodka with soda, or Champagne every now and again will not kill you, but those are exceptions that you can make only when in maintenance mode—not while you're trying to get fit.

My favorite good A would have to be the nutrient-rich powerhouse fruit, **avocado**. It contains oleic acid, a compound in avocados' healthy monounsaturated fats, which may trigger your body to actually quiet hunger (definitely a good thing on the five-day plan).

I also love **alliums** such as garlic, onions, and shallots. Scientists believe the components in onions and garlic called allyl sulfides and

bioflavonoids may help lower blood pressure. They also contain saponins, which may prevent tumors and reduce cholesterol. Quercetin, an anti-inflammatory antioxidant, is an important nutrient found in alliums and may benefit people with inflammatory conditions such as arthritis.

B

Bread is one of those foods you will have to live without during the five days of the plan because it's a processed, refined carbohydrate. Post-program, if you are going to occasionally indulge, make sure the bread is 100 percent whole wheat or multi-grain and has plenty of fiber, but contains no white flour, corn syrup, or sugar. Indulge moderately—one slice, not two. Some of my favorites include a low-carb, high-fiber natural lavash roll-up from a

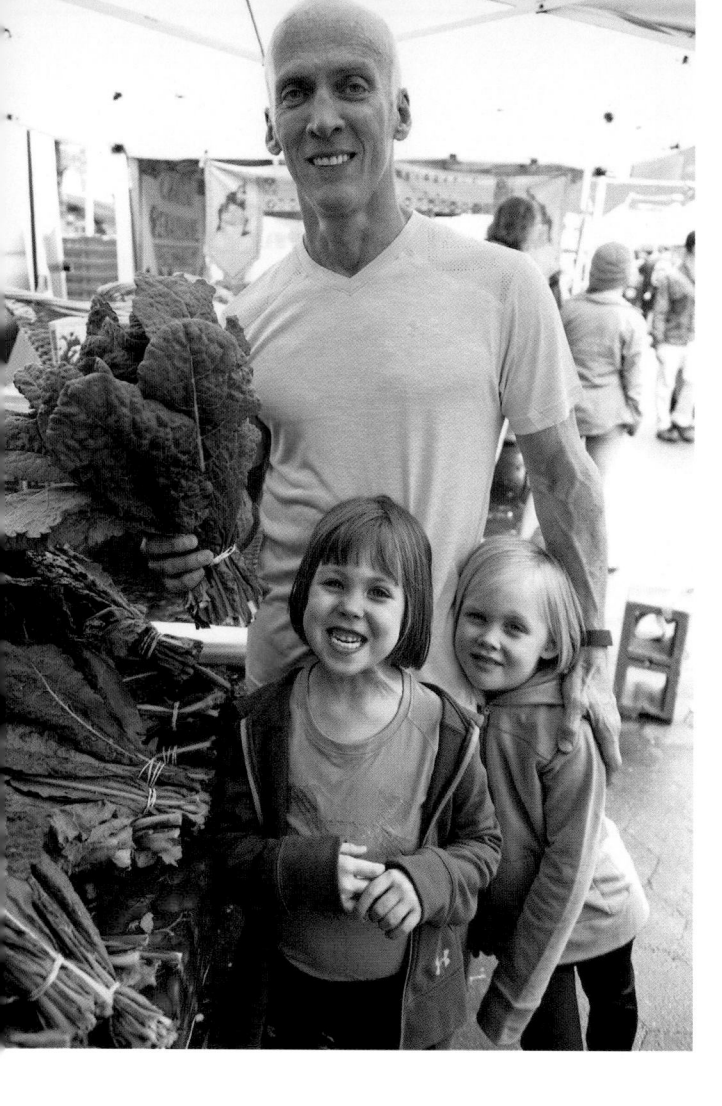

berries. Whether in a fruit salad, atop steel cut oats, or in a breakfast smoothie, they are nutrient, antioxidant, and fiber powerhouses, making them mainstays in our kitchen and our daily nutrition regimen.

And I love **beans**—along with peas and lentils, which are considered legumes—because they are the most versatile and nutritious foods available. They are a superfood, packed with up to sixteen grams of protein along with fifteen grams of fiber and fifteen percent of the recommended daily allowance for complex carbohydrates. Add to that potassium, calcium, magnesium, iron, zinc, folate, and antioxidants. Emilia, Francesca, and I really love eating beans in salads, on vegetable tacos, and in a low-fat homemade hummus (the recipe in on page 198) that the girls gobble up. Beans have an added benefit of loads of soluble fiber, an ingredient that regulates blood sugars and consequently, may help ease mood swings. I must admit, I have tried and tested the mighty bean, and it hasn't yet failed me. My favorite new discovery is a great company called Fig Food Company that sells BPA-free pouches of organic, ready-to-eat beans, allowing you to get your beans quickly and easily when you want them.

C

There isn't anything good to say about processed or refined **carbohydrates**. You will abstain from eating any refined or processed foods during the program. Foods such as french fries, fast food, white bread, and white rice are totally taboo. They are digested too rapidly, leaving you feeling hungry again very quickly. Eating too many of these carbs is one of the main causes of obesity in America.

Vegetables, whole grains, and fruits are the healthy carbohydrates that should be in your daily diet post-program. Emilia, Francesca, and I are

company called Damascus Bakeries and an organic sprouted grain flax bread from Ezekiel.

My favorite Bs are **berries** and **beans**. While only vegetarians can have beans on the five-day plan and you won't eat any berries during that time, berries—strawberries, blueberries, raspberries, and blackberries—are powerful superfoods. They are rich in antioxidants, nutrients, and phytochemicals, which may prevent (and in some cases, reverse) the effects of aging, cardiovascular disease, arthritis, diabetes, high blood pressure, and certain types of cancer. I only eat and serve Emilia and Francesca organic fresh or frozen particularly fond of **cruciferous vegetables** such as cauliflower, broccoli, cabbage, and Brussels sprouts.

D

You're going to abstain from eating **dairy** for the five days of the program.

I am generally anti-dairy, or at least of the school of thought that if consumed, it should be minimal. But if you are not getting swimsuit-ready or trying to squeeze into the skinny jeans, the natural probiotics of yogurt contains an abundant supply of good bacteria for the digestive system. Emilia and Francesca do enjoy two percent plain Greek yogurt, and I serve them two percent organic milk (usually) mixed with almond milk and some liquid vitamins. They also like goat's milk, which I like for its calcium content. The only other dairy they consume is a sprinkle of fresh grated Parmesan cheese and the occasional treat of ice cream or gelato. I serve the girls only organic dairy products.

E

Extra sweeteners and sugars are out. For the duration of the program (and hopefully long-term), you will avoid eating foods with added sugars (most likely the biggest cause of obesity). Also taboo are artificial sweeteners such as Equal, Sweet'N Low, and Splenda, plus Acesulfame potassium (aka Ace K), a commonly used artificial calorie-free sugar substitute. There has been much discussion about which (if any) sweeteners are healthy to use. I have done extensive research and like what I have read and heard about Stevia and Xylitol. I do use these two natural sweeteners in my One-of-a-Kind Supplements® and in baking with Emilia and Francesca.

One of my favorite Es (other than Emilia) is the **egg**. Often maligned and mainly misunderstood, eggs are some of the most nutrient-rich sources of protein, minerals, and amino acids, and they are a staple in my kitchen. As discussed later in this chapter in the sidebar "Debunking Food Myths," the once-thought-evil yolk is not that bad after all.

F

The importance of **fiber** in your daily diet cannot be overstated. It is key to keeping your body regular in weight control in addition to many other health benefits. In a nutshell, fiber—both soluble and insoluble—conveys a feeling of fullness in the stomach as a result of absorbing water. Additionally, if you consume many high-fiber foods, you are likely to eat fewer empty-calorie foods such as solid fats and sweets.

The next F to talk about is **fat**. All fats are not bad. You need them in your diet for your body to function optimally. Essentially, fats from fish, nuts, and vegetable oils are generally healthy. The answer isn't eliminating fat from your diet, it's learning to make healthy choices that cut the bad fats and embrace the good ones. Essentially, you want to avoid trans and saturated fats (often found in many packaged snacks, treats, and sweets). On food labels, look not at total fat content, but at saturated and trans fats.

Lastly, the notion that **fat-free** is healthy is erroneous. Fat-free foods are often higher in sodium and/or sugar, to enhance the flavor lost by omitting fat. The key to optimal health is balancing your calories, good fats, and bad fats with overall calorie consumption. Cut your calorie consumption and increase your calorie expenditure (by moving your body). Eating too much of a "good thing" is not good, and that's the fallacy of the low-fat craze.

G

Though these are a no-no on the five-day part of the plan, consuming foods rich in fiber such as whole **grains** as part of overall healthy eating reduces the risk of coronary heart disease and may reduce constipation. High-fiber foods such as whole grains help provide a feeling of fullness with fewer calories. Selecting whole grains for at least half your daily servings of carbs may help maintain your weight. People who eat whole grains as part of a healthy diet have a reduced risk of some chronic diseases. Grains are also important sources of many nutrients including fiber, B vitamins (e.g., thiamin, riboflavin, niacin, and folate) and minerals (e.g., iron, magnesium, and selenium).

The three below are my favorites. In addition to the basic benefits of grains, they help maintain optimum health due to the phytochemicals they contain, many of which are still being identified. I've included delicious family-friendly recipes for each of these grains in the recipe section of chapter 4.

- **Farro.** This is a dense grain that contains a hefty amount of protein, fiber, and micronutrients.

- **Quinoa.** This is considered a superfood because it contains more protein than any other grain. The protein in quinoa is complete and contains all nine essential amino acids. It is especially high in lysine, methionine, and cysteine. Quinoa is rich in iron, calcium, riboflavin, potassium, vitamin B6, niacin, and thiamin. It's also a good source of magnesium, phosphorous, and folate; high in dietary fiber; and gluten-free.

- **Buckwheat** contains high amounts of immune-boosting zinc, tissue-building copper, and manganese, which protects your bones.

H

Herbs and spices play an important role in my kitchen. Not only are they flavor-enhancing, but they also have an abundant amount of health-boosting properties. I've really enjoyed sharing my passion with Emilia and Francesca. Here are twelve of my favorite herbs and their respective health properties.

Anise (star anise)
The natural flavor of licorice has natural wellness properties. When anyone in my family is congested and battling coldlike symptoms, I put a whole star anise in water with fresh ginger and lemon, steep for thirty to forty-five minutes, pour it into our favorite mugs, and sip it slowly. It definitely speeds up the healing process.

Basil
I would be remiss if I didn't include one of Emilia and Francesca's favorite herbs on this list. Their love affair with basil started out innocently enough with some basil finding its way onto a pizza. They have grown to love it in my homemade tomato sauces and my Tomato-Watermelon Salsa (page 196). Little do they know that it is one of the healthiest herbs. Basil has loads of vitamins A, C, and K, magnesium, iron, potassium, and calcium, as well as antibacterial properties and flavonoids, which protect DNA.

Cayenne pepper
This spice has been known to boost metabolism, and I like to top off my green juice with a sprinkle or two. Additionally, it can act as an anti-irritant to provide relief for upset stomachs, ulcers, sore throats, coughs, and even diarrhea. It can help fight colds and flus by breaking up mucus and prevents some funguses from forming. It's also an anti-allergen and stimulates digestion.

Cinnamon
This spice plays a part in my family's early morning food ritual, as we sprinkle it on our steel-cut oatmeal. Research shows that cinnamon can help regulate blood sugar, which may also minimize the all-too-common mid-morning energy crashes (a.k.a. kiddie meltdown). It's also a great source for the trace mineral manganese, which activates enzymes essential to building bones and metabolizing carbohydrates and fat. Emilia and

Francesca like to sprinkle it on their french toast and in their breakfast smoothies, too. To top it all off, cinnamon is also an excellent source of dietary fiber, iron, and calcium. At best, this combo of calcium and fiber may help reduce the risk of colon cancer and lower cholesterol levels, but at the very least, it can relieve constipation and diarrhea.

Dill

I love using dill in my green juice and to top wild salmon dishes. Not only does it taste wonderful, but it's also packed with calcium, manganese, iron, and flavonoids. In addition to its nutritional qualities, dill can boost your immune system, protect your bones, provide digestive help, and relieve a range of problems including insomnia, diarrhea, dysentery, hiccups, and more.

Garlic

Aside from warding off vampires (you never know where they may lurk), garlic has a multitude of healthful properties. According to the National Library of Medicine, part of the National Institutes of Health, garlic is widely used for several conditions linked to the blood system and heart, including hardening of the arteries, high cholesterol, heart attack, coronary heart disease, and hypertension. For centuries, people have used it to combat colds, and it does boost the immune system. It also contains manganese, vitamins B6 and C, selenium, and fiber.

Ginger

Ginger is known to have more than twelve types of antioxidants, making it useful for treating many disorders. Like other spices, it is used widely for medicinal purposes. It contains essential oils, protein, calcium, phosphorus, iron, vitamin C, choline, folate, inositol, manganese, panthotenic acid, silicon, and a small amount of vitamin B3. I add it to my daily juice and steep it with fresh

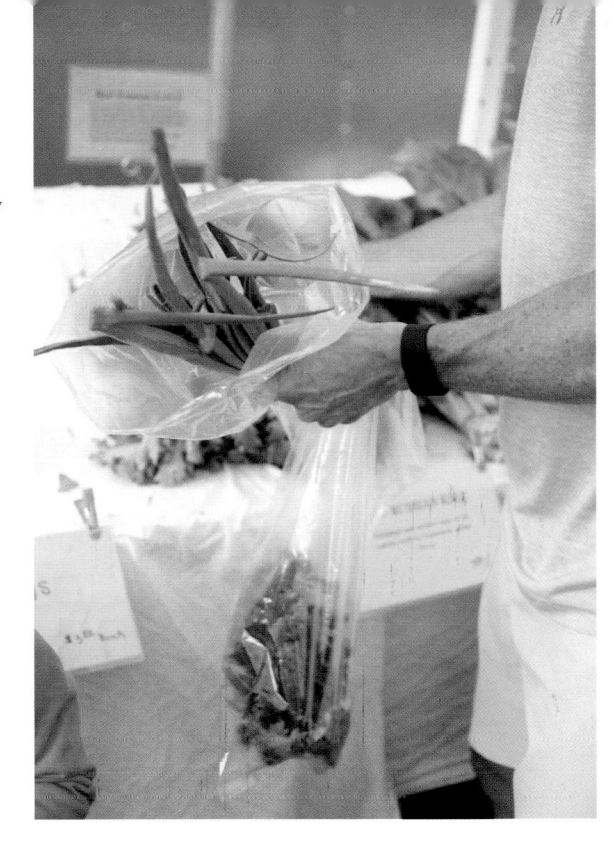

lemon and a bit of honey when I feel under the weather. While researching ginger's healthful benefits, I found that it can help to fight fatigue and muscle soreness (both symptoms I would happily live without). I slice a piece of it into disks and boil it with a big glass of water and a piece of cinnamon bark. I cover it, leave it steeping for about half an hour until it turns golden, pour it in my favorite mug, and sip it slowly. I immediately feel the benefits.

Oregano

One herb I frequently use in my kitchen, oregano contains thirty times more polyphenols than potatoes, twelve times more than oranges, and four times more than blueberries. Polyphenols are great because they act as antioxidants and protect cells against damage caused by free radicals. They also have been associated with cancer prevention and reducing the effects of aging. A tablespoon (4 g) of oregano has as much antioxidant power as a medium-sized apple. It also contains vitamins A, B6, C, E, and K, as well as fiber, folate, iron, magnesium, calcium, and potassium.

Parsley

Parsley provides nature's best carotenoids and is a nutrition powerhouse of a few known anticancer and anti-inflammatory phytonutrients and flavonoids (e.g., lutein, zeaxanthin, apiol, rutin, and apigenin). This tiny-leaf plant is rich in chlorophyll, vitamins A, B, C, and K, folate, and iron. It has high beneficial mineral contents such as calcium, magnesium, manganese, phosphorus, potassium, sodium, vanadium, and zinc. I add it to my green juice every morning. From helping with bad breath to protecting against inflammatory problems such as arthritis, this little green herb is all that and more.

Rosemary

The natural acids present in rosemary help in protecting the body's cells and DNA from free radical damage, and it is also a good source of iron, calcium, and vitamin B6. Along with sage and thyme, rosemary is absolutely essential for cooking my Thanksgiving turkey. You can find the recipe for the perfect roasted turkey breast on page 198.

Sage

Sage may help preserve memory and sooth sore throats. I use lots of fresh sage leaves when I roast my Thanksgiving turkey.

Turmeric

Turmeric is perhaps best known for giving Indian curry its flavor and yellow color. It has been used worldwide for centuries to help with digestion and treat skin diseases and wounds. It contains curcumin, which is a powerful antioxidant that scavenges free radicals in the body, which damage cells, mess with DNA, and can even cause cells to die.

S

Seeds, such as chia, flax, sesame, pumpkin, sunflower, and pomegranate are all nutrient-rich and should be included in your daily diet. You'll also be happy to know they are permissible on the five-day plan.

- Pomegranate seeds are packed with antioxidants and fat-burning vitamin C.

- Hemp seeds are not only complete proteins but are vegetarian and vegan-friendly, too. They contain all twenty known amino acids, including nine essential amino acids our bodies cannot produce, all of which are necessary to building muscle. Sprinkle some in a post-workout shake for a pine nut–like flavor.

- Chia seeds are a great source of bone-building calcium.

- Pumpkin seeds contain iron, which help maintain high energy levels.

- Sesame seeds are great for heart health. The rich seeds contain linoleic acid, an omega-6 fatty acid that may help control harmful cholesterol.

- Flaxseeds, with their nutty flavor, cancer-thwarting lignans compounds, and omega-3 fatty acids, reduce inflammation that can lead to disease.

My favorite company is Navitas. I use their hemp seeds, chia seeds, flax seeds, and cacao nibs. They are readily available in most supermarkets.

Getting the Kiddo Okay

All right, we know how healthful herbs and spices are and how much they enhance the flavor of the foods we eat, but how do we get our children to try them? Emilia and Francesca embraced them warily at first, save the dash of pepper here and there. They are both very tactile, so when I take them shopping, they touch everything in sight. First, I allowed them to gently touch a basil leaf between their fingers, and they loved the smell. Next was rosemary, followed by dill and parsley. It's often very simple for kids: If it doesn't feel slimy or smell "yucky," it passes "the touch and smell test" and can make its way onto the table.

I make sure to keep plenty of fresh organic herbs in the kitchen, ensuring at least one will end up in that day's meals. To date, the girls have tried each of the herbs on the previous list at least once. Their palates are a lot more sophisticated than mine was at five years old.

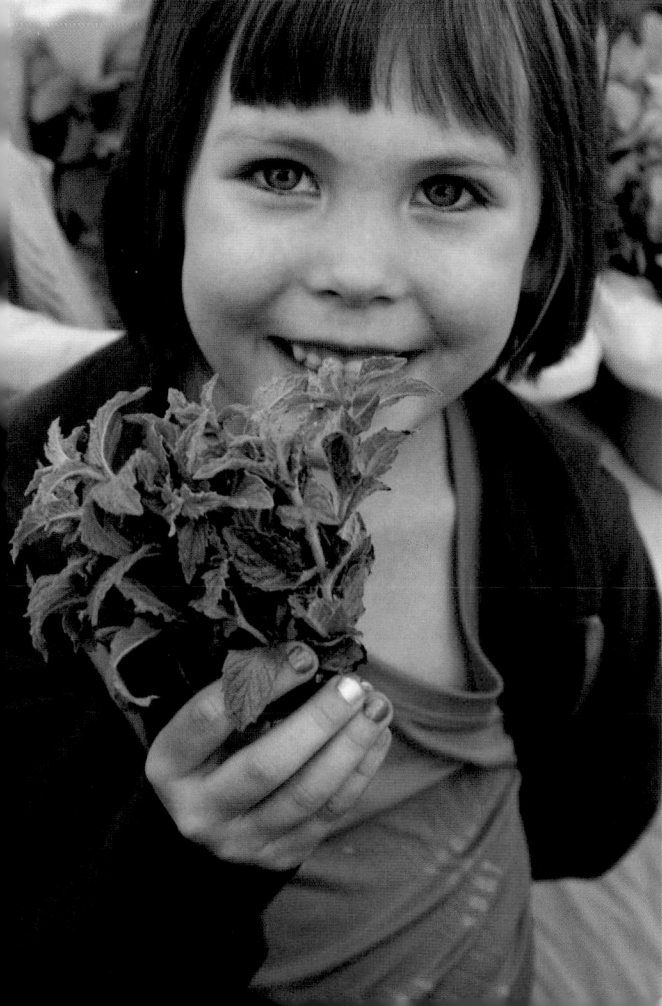

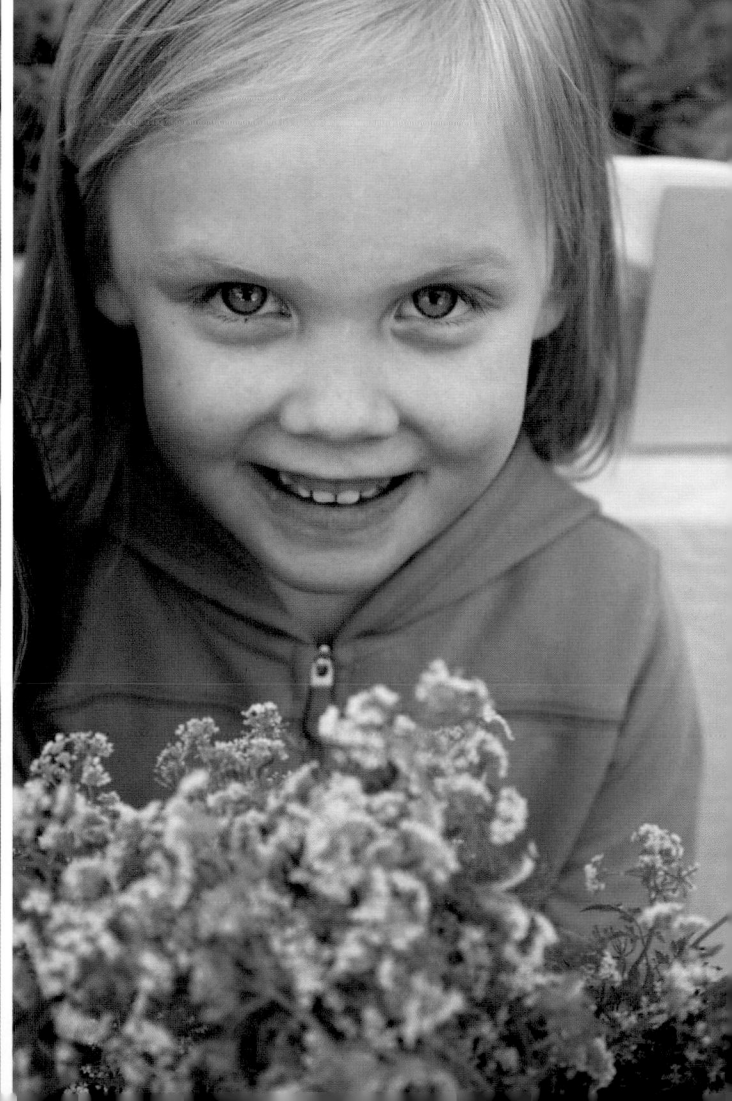

DEBUNKING FOOD AND NUTRITION MYTHS

There are a lot of great foods out there that get a bad rep. I'm here to clear up some misconceptions about some really good foods.

Watermelon

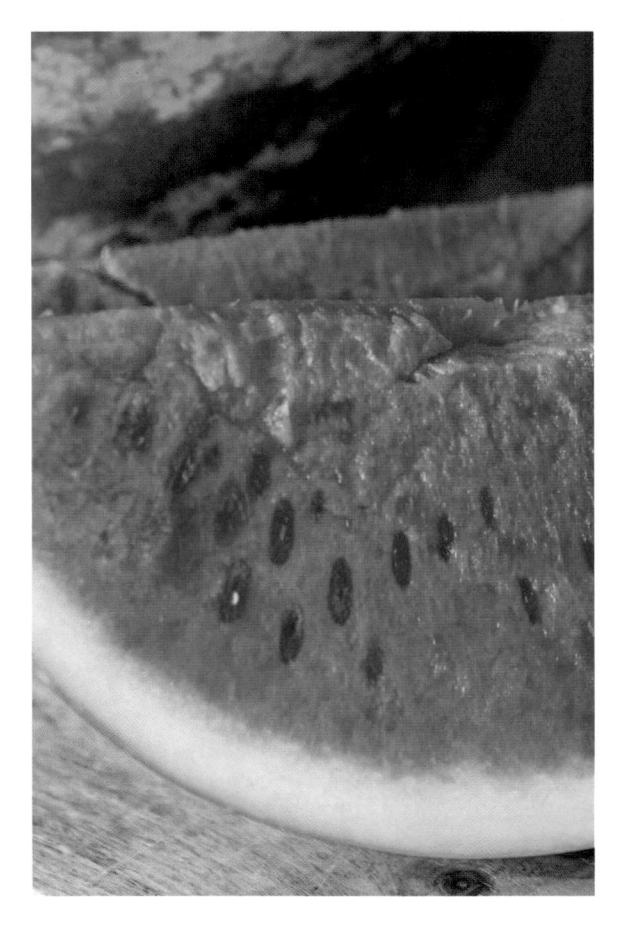

Despite popular belief that watermelon is made up of only water and sugar, watermelon is actually considered a nutrient-dense food, a food that provides a high amount of vitamins, minerals, and antioxidants for a low amount of calories. Its refreshing quality and sweet taste help combat the heat and also provide a guilt-free, low maintenance dessert for kids and adults alike. I have actually used it in a delicious tomato-basil salad and its refreshing taste and crunch turned another "hum drum" salad into something exciting. If you're still not convinced, check out the nutritional breakdown for one cup (150 grams) of watermelon:

- It contains just 43 calories and 0 grams of fat.

- It provides seventeen percent of the vitamin A, twenty-one percent of the vitamin C, two percent of the iron, and one percent of the calcium recommended for daily nutrition.

- Watermelon also has thiamin, riboflavin, niacin, vitamin B6, folate, pantothenic acid, magnesium, phosphorus, potassium, zinc, copper, manganese, selenium, choline, lycopene, and betaine.

- It has more lycopene than any other fruit or vegetable, according to The National Watermelon Promotion Board.

- It is made up of ninety-two percent water, making it super hydrating.

What's more refreshing in the summer heat than a juicy watermelon? I would have to say that watermelon is the go-to fruit for Emilia and Francesca after a day outdoors in the summer, whether on the beach or at the carousel. Watermelon hydrates and energizes while scintillating the taste buds.

Avocado

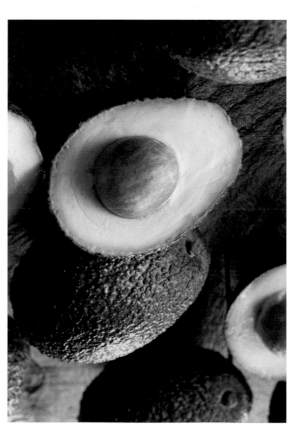

Avocado is one of my favorite fruits. Emilia, Francesca, and I love avocado in salads, smoothies and, as you will see in the recipe section, with my delicious Roasted Turkey Avocado Salad (page 162) and Tuna Spinach Bowl (page 173). But this very tasty, nutrient-rich food contains more fat and calories than more popular fruits such as berries. So is it healthy to eat on a regular basis? See for yourself:

- Avocados provide twenty essential nutrients including eight essential vitamins: vitamins B6, C, E, and K, folate, thiamin, riboflavin, and pantothenic acid.

- Avocados serve as a good source of essential minerals including potassium and magnesium,

yet contain no sodium, which contributes to their heart-healthy status.

- Avocados contain 81 micrograms per ounce (28 g) of the phytochemical lutein, which helps maintain healthy eyes and skin. In addition to being a rich source of nutrients, avocados also function as nutrient-boosters by helping the body absorb essential fat-soluble nutrients.

- A medium-sized avocado contains approximately 20 to 25 grams of fat. This high fat content caused many to shy away from eating avocados in the mid-1980s when nutritionists emphasized low-fat foods. Recent guidelines from the American Heart Association (AHA) stress the importance of the type of fat you consume, noting the differences between the good fats found in vegetables, or unsaturated fats, and the fats that contribute to high blood cholesterol levels, known as saturated and trans fats (see the earlier sidebar, "Good Fats versus Bad Fats"). The AHA recommends that your total fat intake should amount to twenty-five to thirty-five percent of your daily calories with saturated fats limited to less than seven percent of those calories and trans fats less than one percent. Avocados contain mostly unsaturated fats, with only about 2 grams of saturated fat and 0 grams of trans fat in a one-ounce (28 g) serving. This makes avocados a part of a heart-healthy diet.

- Avocados are also a great source of fiber. According to The Proceedings of the Florida State Horticultural Society, each one-ounce serving has 2 grams soluble fiber and almost 3 grams insoluble. Eating fiber helps regulate bowel movements, lowers blood cholesterol levels, and evens out blood sugar.

- Avocados, when eaten every day (especially to replace bad fats), can help lower bad cholesterol and even decrease the risk of heart disease.

Eggs

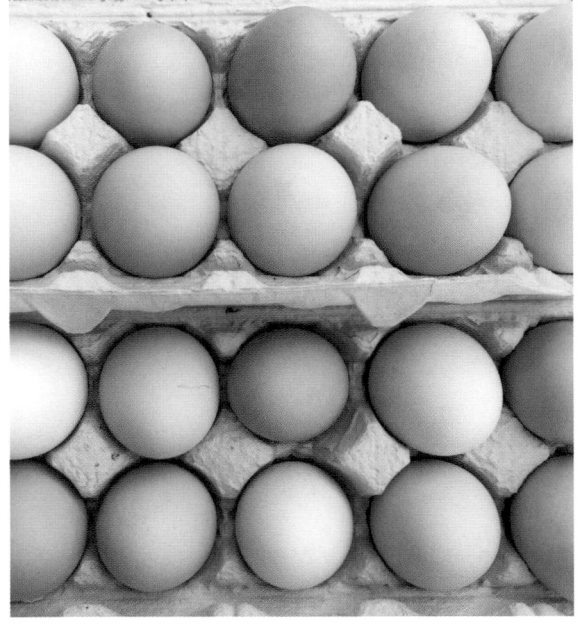

Way back in the day when I was training and competing in natural bodybuilding shows, I would consume three to four dozen eggs a week. Of course, old school beliefs held that the egg whites (i.e., albumin) contained all the protein while the yolks contained the fat. But recent research has debunked that myth and given the much-maligned egg yolk the reprieve it rightfully deserves.

- A whole egg contains 7 grams of protein.

- The yolk contains half the protein and most of the vitamins and minerals. Yes, the yolks have cholesterol, but unless you have a history of high cholesterol or heart disease, they won't affect your cholesterol levels.

- Whole eggs are practically a perfect food. They are chock full of almost every essential vitamin and mineral, including vitamin D (one of the few foods that has it), omega-3 fatty acids, vitamins B6 and B12, riboflavin, folate, and choline. And those vitamin Bs are actually

believed to help ward off heart disease.

- The amino acid L-arginine in eggs is vital to producing protein and releasing growth hormones.

- Whole eggs are power foods, one of my MVPs (most valuable protein sources). But when I'm watching fats and calories, I mix egg whites and whole eggs for my frittatas and other egg dishes.

- Eggs make a great snack. If you're watching your calories, I recommend hard-boiling three to six eggs in the morning and leaving them on the kitchen counter at home or bringing them to the office.

Nuts

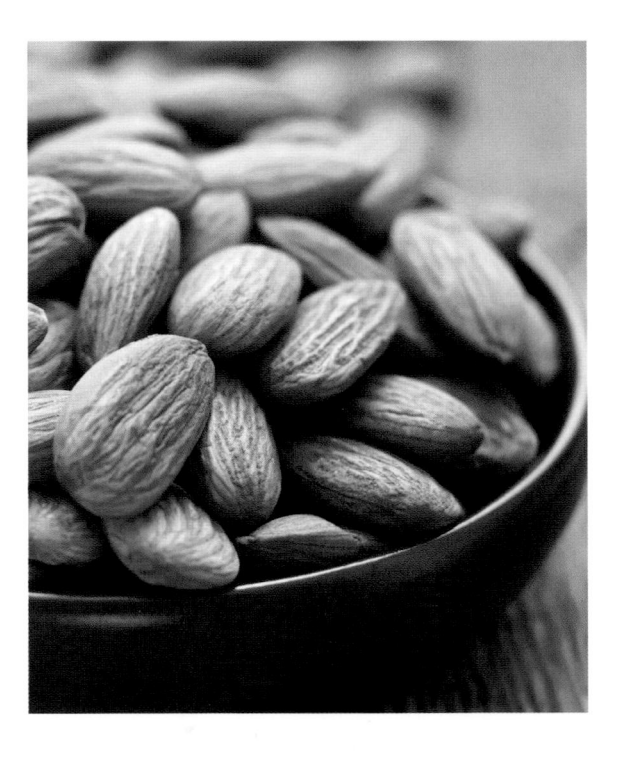

Nuts have gotten a bad rap because of their high fat content. But their protein, heart-healthy fats, high fiber, and antioxidant content earn them a place in your daily diet. I often say "less is more,"

and portion control is key to healthfully enjoying nuts. See the list below for my favorite nuts and their respective nutritional breakdown:

- **Almonds.** These nuts make it to the top of the list. One ounce (approximately 23 nuts or 28 g) contains 160 calories, 6 grams of protein, 6 grams of carbs, and 4 grams of fiber. Compared to other nuts, they contain the most fiber—about 3 grams per ounce (28 g)—and are the richest in vitamin E, a powerful antioxidant. They also contain magnesium, calcium, and potassium and are high in monounsaturated fats. Emilia, Francesca, and I love making fresh ground almond butter and enjoy it as a snack on celery and apples, in smoothies, and in our morning oatmeal.

- **Walnuts.** These nuts are another one of my favorites. One ounce (approximately 14 halves or 28 g) contains 190 calories, 4 grams of protein, 4 grams of carbs, and 2 grams of fiber. They are a great source of potassium, magnesium, calcium, and selenium. They contain the most antioxidants and are the richest in omega-3 fatty acids of any nuts. As an aside, they contain manganese, which may reduce PMS symptoms. I personally use walnuts in some of my sauteed vegetable dishes and am a huge fan of walnut oil.

- **Pistachio nuts.** One ounce (approximately 49 nuts or 28 g) contains 160 calories, 4 grams of protein, 8 grams of carbs, and 3 grams of fiber. They are great source of potassium, phosphorous, calcium, and magnesium. I love the whole process of opening the shell and munching on them when I am writing late at night. Plus, the pile of shells keeps me mindful of how many I've eaten.

- **Pine nuts.** One ounce (approximately 165 nuts or 28 g) contains 190 calories, 4 grams of protein, 4 grams of carbs, and 1 gram of fiber. They are a good source of plant-derived nutrients, essential minerals, vitamins, and heart-healthy monounsaturated fatty acids that help reduce cholesterol levels in blood. I like to use them in my healthy pesto sauces and toast them with roasted vegetable dishes.

- **Cashews.** One ounce (approximately 18 nuts or 28 g) contains 165 calories, 5 grams of protein, 8.5 grams of carbs, and 1 gram of fiber. They are brainpower boosters and are rich in iron and zinc (great for your immune system and oxygenating your cells) and magnesium, which may improve memory and protect against age-related memory loss.

- **Brazil nuts.** One ounce (approximately 6 nuts or 28 g) contains 185 calories, 4 grams of protein, 3 grams of carbs, and 2 grams of fiber. Just one Brazil nut packs more than 100 percent of the daily value for the mineral selenium, which may help prevent certain cancers including bone, prostate, and breast cancer. High levels of selenium can be harmful, so stick to a serving or less.

- **Hazelnuts.** One ounce (approximately 21 nuts or 28 g) contains 180 calories, 4 grams of protein, 5 grams of carbs, and 3 grams of fiber. They are heart-healthy and packed with folate, manganese, and copper.

CHILDHOOD VEGGIES REVISITED

Baked potatoes, corn on the cob, and iceberg lettuce—these are just some of the staples that loaded the vegetable bin in the refrigerator in my childhood house. Were they good? Were they bad? Did they have any nutritional value at all? Here's the latest on their relative healthfulness.

White Potatoes

These are healthy, containing 5 grams of fiber, 4 grams of protein, ten percent of your daily iron, twenty percent of your daily potassium, and seventy percent of your vitamin C. They're also known to fight hypertension. Make sure to eat the skin—my favorite part—and lose the pat of butter and dollop of sour cream. Do you like french fries? They're definitely a favorite in my house. I love my kitchen gadgets, and I discovered a quick and healthy way to enjoy them. ActiFry by T-Fal is an air fryer that uses just one tablespoon (15 ml) of oil and in thirty minutes makes delicious and healthy fries. Roasted baked potatoes are also my go-to post-workout snack.

Iceberg Lettuce

Growing up on Long Island in the sixties, I ate salad with most meals and iceberg lettuce starred in those, along with cucumbers, bell peppers, and celery. When I graduated college in 1982 and moved to New York City, I was brainwashed into thinking that iceberg lettuce was devoid of any nutrients. But iceberg has made a comeback. Heck, the world-famous Palm Restaurant never gave up on the iceberg wedge, albeit with a large serving of blue cheese atop. The fact is that iceberg lettuce contains nearly twenty percent of your daily dose of vitamin K and fifteen percent of your daily dose of vitamin A.

Corn

Grilled corn on the cob is the quintessential summer barbecue fare. Its bad rap is due to guilt-by-association with high-fructose corn syrup, a sweetener made from corn that has had all the nutrition and fiber processed out of it. One ear of corn has four grams of fiber (fifteen percent of the amount you need in a day). It also has more than twenty-five percent of the recommended daily allowance for the mineral thiamin, which helps cells convert carbohydrates from food into energy. Lastly, it also contains zeaxanthin and lutein, plant chemicals that help keep your eyes healthy.

MY TOP TEN SUPERFOODS

The *Oxford English Dictionary* states that a superfood is "a nutrient-rich food considered especially beneficial for health and well-being." When thinking about which foods make the list for me, I considered this: What are the foods that I rely on, and what are the foods that my daughters and I go to on a regular basis to keep us healthy and energized for our fast-paced, full lives? As a single father of twin girls, I depend on and refer to this list regularly to ensure that we are optimally fueled. Here are my favorite superfoods, in no special order.

If a superfood is okay for the five-day plan, you'll see this icon: 5. If it's not, you'll see this: 5.

If it's okay only for vegetarians, you'll see this: ❚.

2% Plain Greek Yogurt

Thicker and creamier than regular yogurt, Greek yogurt is higher in calcium than some other dairy products and packed full of protein. A seven-ounce (200 g) container has two to three times the amount of protein (a whopping 20 g) and less sugar than regular yogurt. The probiotics in Greek yogurt can help with digestion, contain loads of good bacteria, and boost immunity. Emilia and Francesca like to add raspberries, blueberries, strawberries, and gluten-free, low-sugar, low-sodium granola to their morning yogurt. "Dairy foods contain practically every nutrient you need for total nutrition—and in just the right balance," says bone health expert, Robert Heaney, M.D. "No other food group in the diet is as complete or as economical." Note: Make sure all your dairy says "organic," or at least "hormone-," "antibiotic-," and "pesticide-free."

Eggs

They are a nutritious, versatile, economical way to fill up on quality protein. "Studies show if you eat eggs at breakfast, you may eat fewer calories during the day and lose weight without significantly affecting cholesterol levels," says Elizabeth Ward, M.S., R.D., author of *The Pocket Idiot's Guide to the New Food Pyramids*. Eggs also contain twelve vitamins and minerals, including choline, which is good for brain development and memory. I enjoy my eggs in a variety of ways: medium-boiled, poached, scrambled, and in frittatas, to name a few.

I started Emilia and Francesca on eggs before they were a year old, splitting one scrambled egg between them. Suddenly at age two, they stopped eating them that way. I do manage to use them in my turkey burger recipes, whole-wheat almond pancakes, and one of their favorites, the occasional treat, french toast.

In the late eighties and nineties, whole eggs—especially the yolks—were shunned because people believed the yolk held all the fat and cholesterol. That may be true, but unless you have a family history of heart disease or cholesterol problems, the yolk's on you—or should be in you. The egg yolk contains a majority of the vitamins and nutrients in the egg. Starting with vitamin A (244 IU), vitamin D (18 IU), calcium (22 mg), folate (25 mg), and ever-important omega-3s (39 mg), eggs are by far my MVP (most valuable protein). One final note about eggs: I do use a ratio of one whole egg to two egg whites when cooking and eating them. I also buy organic, free-range eggs. They don't necessarily need to be organic, but they should be hormone- and pesticide-free.

5 Berries

Berries pack an incredible amount of nutritional goodness into a small package. They are loaded with antioxidants and phytonutrients, low in calories, and high in water and fiber to help control blood sugar and keep you full longer. For my clients with an incurable sweet tooth, I recommend washing and freezing berries. When the urge for something sweet arises, feast on one of the frozen treats; it's not exactly a candy bar, but a lot healthier, and without the fat, calories, or added sugar.

Which berry is healthiest? They are all nutrient-rich, but each one has unique health benefits. One cup (145 g) of strawberries has more vitamin C than an orange and has strong immune-boosting properties. Blueberries are full of powerful antioxidants and, research has indicated, links to good vision, acuity, and brain development. Raspberries, at seven grams of fiber, have more fiber than a bran muffin. They are also rich in antioxidants and are heart-healthy. Blackberries, lowest in calories at just 43 calories for a one-cup (145 g) serving, are an excellent source of fiber and vitamin C. Additionally, the berry's striking dark color comes from anthocyanin, a powerful phytonutrient that may protect from diseases such as cancer.

I know I've said a lot about the importance of eating organic foods. In my opinion, this is especially true when referring to berries. Here, pesticides are sprayed directly onto the fruit, and even with washing the fruit, which you should do with all fruits before eating, it is likely pesticide residue will remain on the fruit. In winter, when organic berries are not in season, I opt for frozen organic berries.

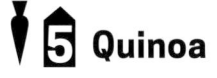 Quinoa

This tiny grain-like seed is a nutritional powerhouse. One cooked cup (185 g) contains eight grams of protein, five grams of fiber, iron, plenty of zinc, vitamin E, and selenium to help control weight and lower risk for heart disease and diabetes. Additionally, it is one of the few grains that provides all nine essential amino acids. Personally, I love its versatility and ease of preparation. I like to toss it in dark green salads with nuts and avocado for those nights when Emilia, Francesca, and I go meatless.

5 Nuts

As I said earlier in the book, nuts are often frowned upon due to their high fat content. But the good far outweighs the bad here. They are a solid source of protein and heart-healthy fats and are high in fiber and antioxidants, vitamins, and minerals. They key to eating nuts is a philosophy I set forth in my first book, "Less is more." For example, twenty-three almonds weighs in at 191 calories. As far as nuts go, almonds were my first love. My girls and I snack on them, roast and cook with them, and are totally addicted to fresh-ground almond butter. To fuel up for my workouts, I often take a tablespoon (16 g) of almond butter with an apple or pear. Walnuts are also a favorite and a great source of vitamin E, selenium, and magnesium. I also love to saute vegetables with walnut oil, and on occasion, use it in salad dressings. Pistachios are my go-to nuts when I am chained to my computer. They are loaded with plant sterols and potassium (a one-ounce [28 g] serving has almost as much potassium as a small banana). The added step of cracking the shell keeps you mindful of and accountable for how much you consume.

Whether you prefer almonds, walnuts, pistachios, or one of the other nuts I previously mentioned, a single serving will satisfy your craving, leaving you sated and nutritionally fortified. Nuts are a staple in Emilia and Francesca's after-school snack bags and tennis bags. Note: Only eat raw or dry-roasted, unsalted nuts to avoid unnecessary fat and sodium.

5 Broccoli

Broccoli is said to be one of America's favorite vegetables—one of Emilia and Francesca's, too. It tastes great, is readily available year-round, is high in soluble and insoluble fiber, and is a rich source of vitamins A, B-complex, C, and K, iron, zinc, phosphorus, and phytonutrients. The girls and I steam it, roast it, grill it, and saute it in stir-fry.

I try to only eat organic broccoli (fresh or frozen). However, in the past couple of years, I have discovered many farmers who aren't certified organic but who do not use any chemicals or pesticides on their produce and fruits. I will choose one of these local farmers over organic produce from another part of the country or world. So if you have a local farmers' market, ask around and see what the local growers are doing.

I know I am cheating a little, but I'm going to add spinach here, too. Look, where would Popeye and Olive Oyl be if it weren't for power of spinach? This powerhouse vegetable is loaded. It's an excellent source of vitamins A (in the form of carotenoids), B2, B6, C, E, and K, manganese, folate, magnesium, iron, copper, calcium, and potassium. It is a very good source of dietary fiber, phosphorus, vitamin B1, zinc, protein, and choline.

5 Salmon

Salmon made the list because of its heart-healthy omega-3 fatty acid content. That's why the American Heart Association recommends eating fatty fish such as salmon twice weekly. Salmon is low in calories (three ounces [85 g] is just 200 calories) and saturated fats and is a good source of protein, potassium, and vitamins B6 and B12. I like to sear it on my cast-iron skillet and serve it rare "sushi style," grill it, or make my newly discovered Crispy Salmon Nuggets (see page 177 for the recipe). Whether for lunch or dinner, salmon is a rich, versatile, nutrient-rich protein that my family and I love to prepare and eat. Note: I only buy wild salmon, and it has to pass my "smell test." I don't want to smell my fish way over in the produce department. With few exceptions, fresh fish doesn't smell fishy.

Beans

Beans are heart-healthy and loaded with insoluble fiber, which helps lower cholesterol, as well as soluble fiber, which promotes digestive health and relieves constipation. They contain no cholesterol, lots of complex carbohydrates, and little fat. In addition, beans are a good source of B vitamins, potassium, and fiber. Eating beans may help prevent colon cancer and reduce blood cholesterol, a leading cause of heart disease.

Emilia and Francesca love edamame, which is loaded with omega-3 fatty acids. Many of my vegetarian clients substitute beans for meat or poultry as their entree, but I also use them as side dishes, in salads, soups, and turkey chili. Note: The U.S. Dietary Guidelines recommend three cups (675 g) of beans weekly. Most of us don't have the time to use dry beans and opt for the convenience of canned beans. When buying canned beans, read the ingredients label to see that there's no added sugar, excessive amounts of sodium, or artificial ingredients. Further, before you use canned beans, thoroughly rinse them in water, which will remove up to forty-five percent of the sodium content. When adding to soups, stews, or turkey chili, add rinsed canned beans for the final ten minutes of cooking. Canned beans are also more convenient to add to cold salads.

If you have the time and patience to use dried beans, follow these necessary steps. With the exception of black-eyed peas, all dried beans must be soaked before they're cooked. Soaking and cooking times vary by bean type, with most needing six to eight hours of soaking and one to two hours of cooking. Many bean varieties,

including kidney beans, naturally contain toxic compounds that are destroyed with proper preparation—soaked beans must boil for at least ten minutes of their lengthy cooking time. Slow-cooked beans not brought to a boil can retain their toxicity and cause food poisoning. I know this sounds rather complicated and, in the case of dried beans, time consuming. About a year ago, I discovered the Fig Food Co., a company that sells ready-to-eat organic beans of every variety in BPA-free pouches. The beans taste fresh, firm, and delicious, are low in sodium (10 mg), and are incredibly user-friendly.

Cauliflower

Cauliflower is a sentimental favorite of mine. I'll never forget taking three-year-old Emilia and Francesca to Whole Foods. I had just picked them up from nursery school and we were shopping for dinner. I told them they could each get one item for dinner. Emilia headed straight to the cauliflower and asked me if it was organic.

Our favorite way to prepare cauliflower is to cut it up in florets, add a little olive oil, salt, and black pepper, and roast or saute until golden and delicious. For added health benefits and flavor, I add turmeric. Cauliflower is packed with vitamins B6, C, and K, as well as folate, choline, dietary fiber, omega-3 fatty acids, manganese, phosphorus, and biotin. It also contains cancer-fighting compounds shown to have anticarcinogenic properties.

Sweet Potatoes

Sweet potatoes are an amazing source of nutritional necessities. One medium potato has more than four times your daily vitamin A needs, plus lots of vitamins B6 and C, potassium, manganese, and fiber. They are also a great source of the antioxidant beta-carotene, which may reduce the risk of certain types of cancer, protect against asthma and heart disease, and postpone aging and degeneration. They do have more natural sugars than other potatoes, but they are also more nutritious and contain fewer calories.

I love everything about roasting and devouring sweet potatoes. Emilia and Francesca enjoy them this way, but they also like healthy air fries. I know healthy fries sound like an oxymoron, but I have a great air fryer from T-Fal. I cut up one or two sweet potatoes add a tablespoon (15 ml) of grapeseed oil, salt, and black pepper. Thirty minutes later, you have perfect, healthy fries without the fat and extra calories.

Five Kid-Friendly Superfoods

Emilia and Francesca have grown up surrounded by healthy foods. I am raising them to understand the importance of good, sound nutrition; to listen to their bellies in determining their level of hunger; and above all, to believe that food is life sustaining, not a reward, consolation, or something to be taken for granted. We don't always eat perfectly, but we make the best choices of what is available. I thought I would add a few items to Emilia and Francesca's kid-friendly superfoods list that we eat pretty much on a regular basis.

1. Oatmeal made the list because of its abundant nutrient content. High in fiber, antioxidants, and tons of other nutrients, oatmeal has been a staple of our breakfast table since the girls were about fifteen months old. It's that hot meal mom always wanted us to have before we started our day—and she was right. It keeps blood glucose stable, which allows kids to focus for longer in school. Research has also shown that oatmeal can help lower cholesterol, aid in digestion and even improve metabolism. We like to add fresh ground cinnamon, berries, and one teaspoon (5 g) of fresh ground almond butter to our breakfast oatmeal.

2. Kiwi, one of Francesca's favorite fruits, is thankfully becoming more readily available across the country, as kiwi from California has started showing up in the produce section at Whole Foods on the East Coast. For a small fruit, it packs a powerful nutrient punch. Kiwis are fat-free and low in calories, provide tons of energy, fiber, and antioxidants, and are packed with vitamins and minerals such as vitamins C and E, potassium, magnesium, lutein, folate, and zinc.

3. Watermelon—I've previously spoken to the health attributes of everyone's favorite summer fruit. I happily serve watermelon to Emilia and Francesca whenever I can find organic melons. This guilt-free pleasure is low in sugar and high in vitamins A and C. It is the perfect low-calorie snack. Studies suggest that for adults, watermelon could also potentially lower blood pressure and reduce the risk of cardiovascular disease.

4. Avocado is an easy choice as one of Emilia and Francesca's superfoods; it was the first fresh fruit they ate when they were about nine months old. Oh how they loved (and still do) the taste and creamy texture. They are the perfect superfood for children because their bodies easily burn the monounsaturated fat so prevalent in avocados. Additionally, kids use the fat for growth, including brain development and eye health. I like to use avocado in salads, wraps, guacamole, and smoothies. The possibilities are endless.

5. Tomatoes contain lots of potassium, fiber, and vitamin C. I like to use them in salads, tomato sauces, and frittatas. They are also a great source of lycopene, which is thought to protect the skin against harmful ultraviolet rays, prevent certain cancers, and lower cholesterol.

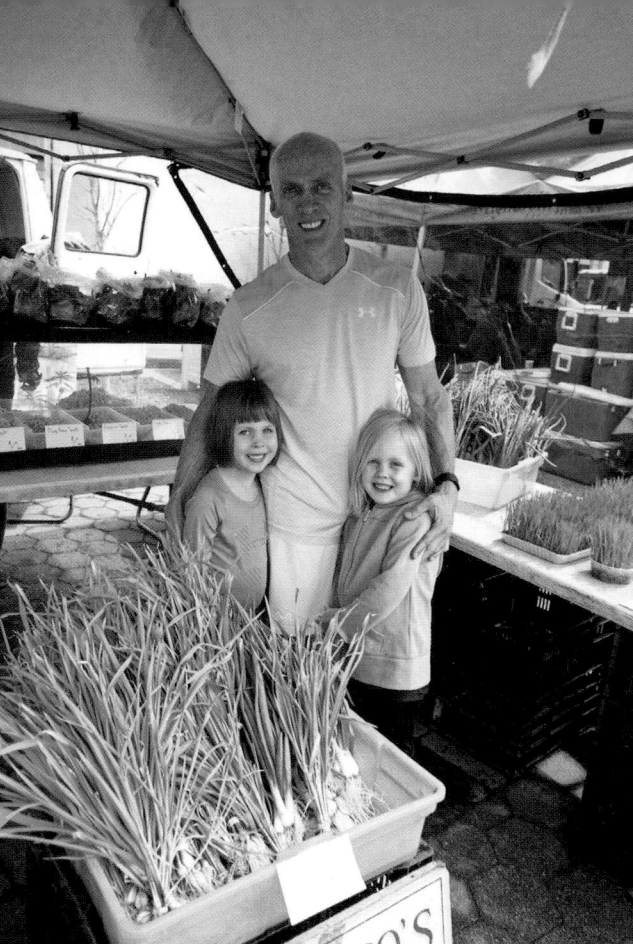
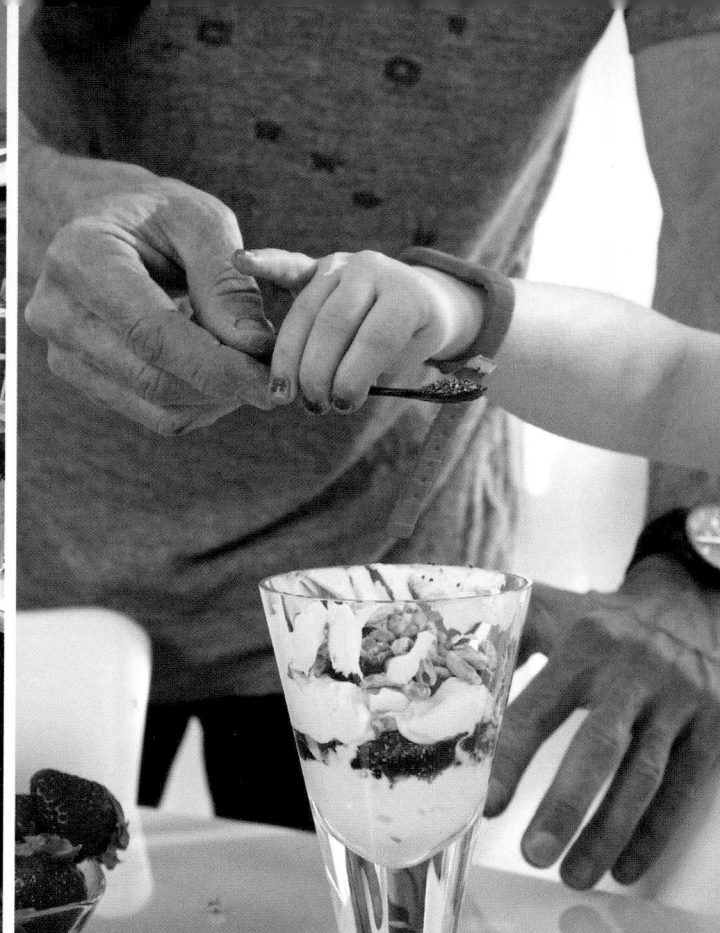

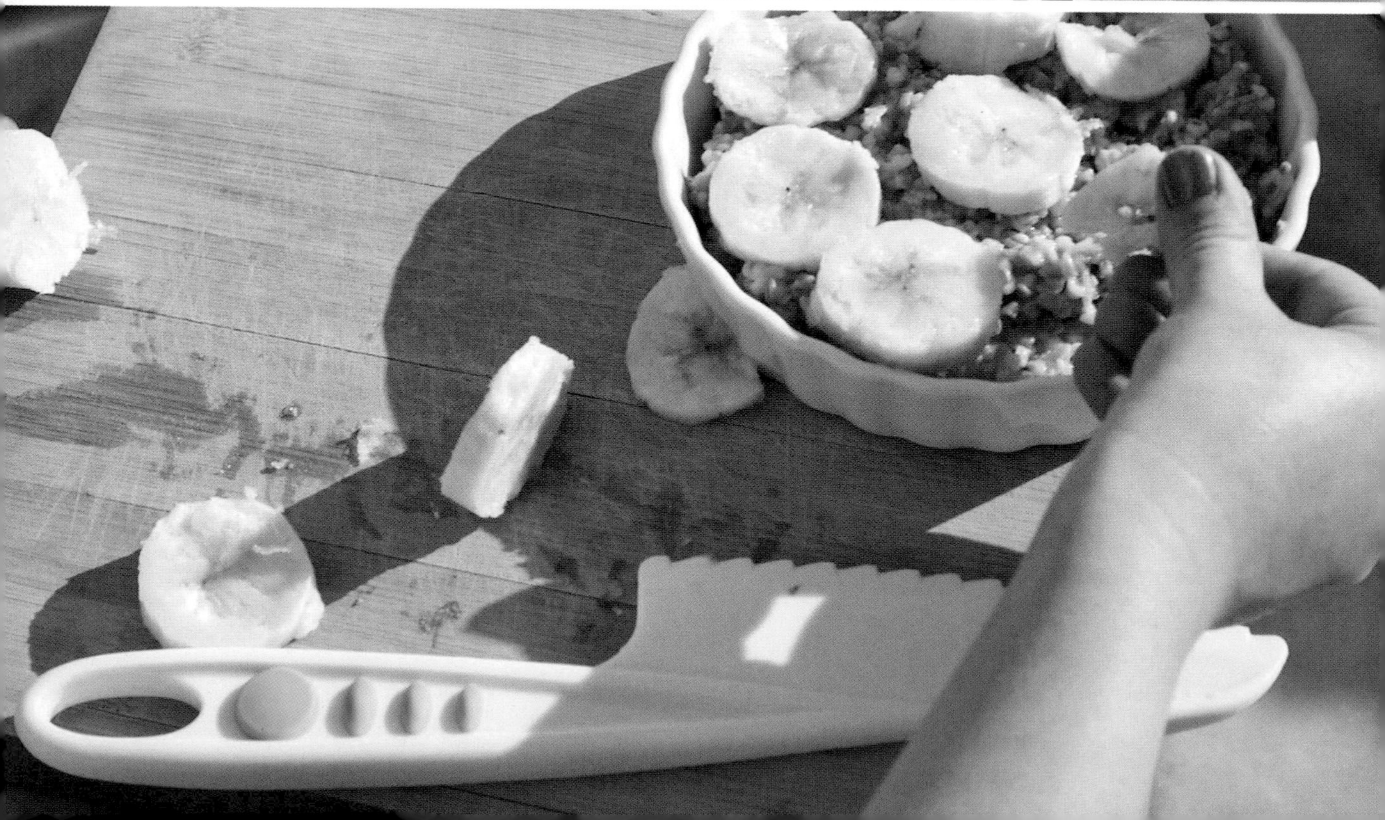

Chapter 4

COOKING WITH YOUR KIDS

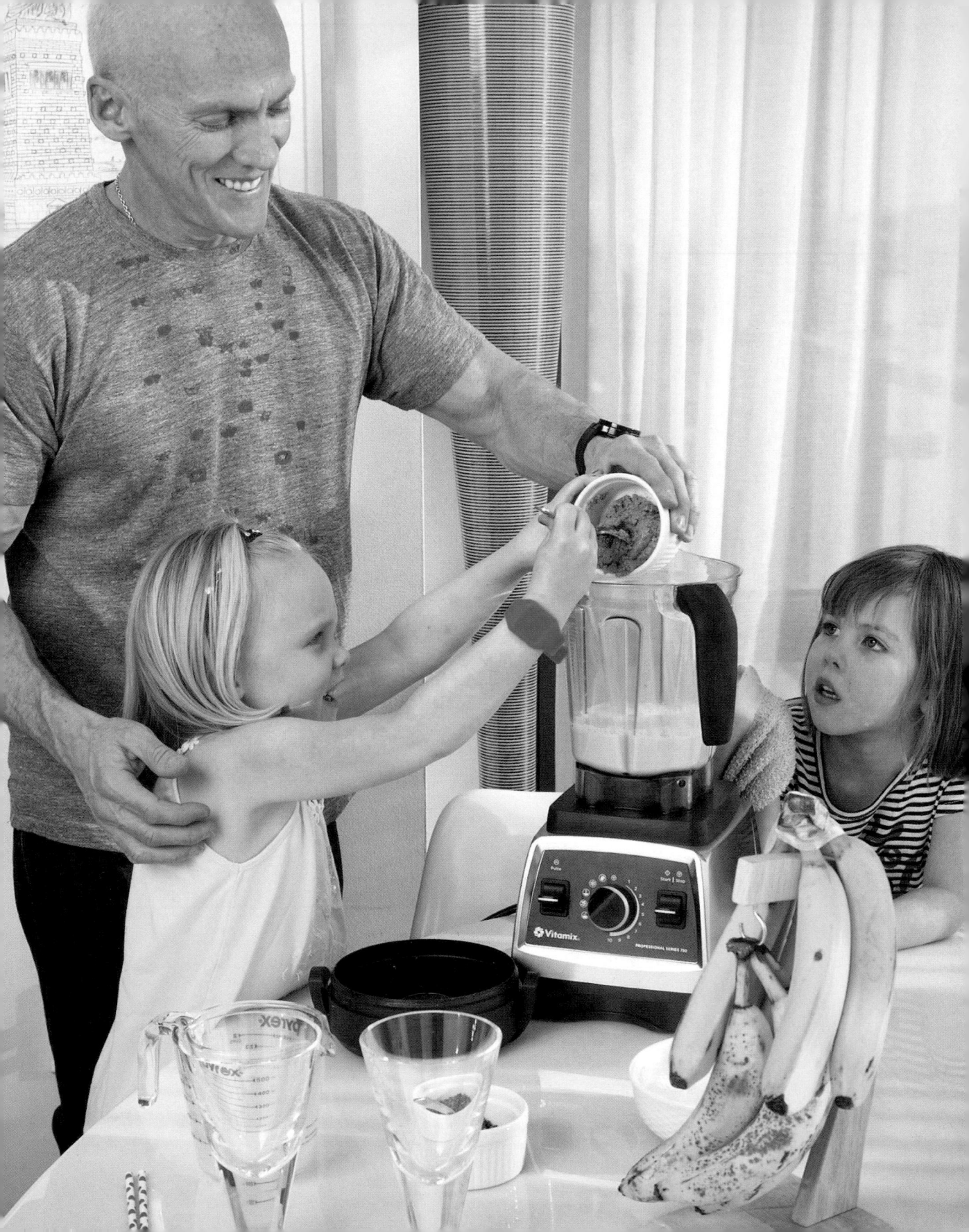

We've talked about the different types of movement and exercise you and your family will incorporate into your life, and now it's time for me to share some of my family's favorite recipes. Consistent with the philosophy of this book, the recipes are easy to prepare, contain about five ingredients each, and take no longer than fifteen minutes from start to finish. They are short on prep time, but big on taste and nutritional value.

While all of the recipes are delicious and nutritious, not all of them are permissible on the five-day plan. For those recipes, you will see one of two symbols: **5** the five-day okay symbol and **15** the vegetarians-only five-day okay symbol, indicating the use of grain and proteins only permissible on the five-day plan for vegetarians. Now get ready to titillate your taste buds as you continue on the path to becoming the Ultimate Wellness Family.

SMOOTHIES AND JUICES

These awesome drinks are great for breakfast or a snack on the run and will keep you and your family charged all morning long. They are fast and easy to make, too. Just put all the ingredients in a blender and go. My blender of choice is the Vitamix 750. It's powerful, versatile (smoothies, hot and cold soups), kid-friendly, and easy to clean up. (See Resources section, page 217, for my favorite products and gadgets.)

BANANA CHOCOLATE PROTEIN SMOOTHIE

This smoothie is sure to satisfy your sweet tooth while fortifying you with potassium, probiotics, and lots of healthy antioxidants.

½ cup (120 ml) of almond milk

1 frozen banana

¼ cup (60 g) low-fat plain Greek yogurt

2 teaspoons (6 g) Navitas cacao nibs (or a comparable brand)

1 tablespoon (16 g) fresh-ground almond butter

Ice, to taste

▸ YIELD: SERVES 1

AVOCADO BERRY SMOOTHIE

Berries, avocado, and mango—it's delicious, nutritious, and energizing.

½ cup (120 ml) almond milk

1 whole avocado

1 lime, juiced

3 cups (765 g) frozen strawberries

1⅓ cups (280 g) frozen chopped mango

▸ YIELD: SERVES 1

BERRY PROTEIN BLAST

I love this appetite-satisfying protein smoothie with its powerful combination of nutrient-rich blackberries, superfood chia seeds, and whey protein powder.

¾ cup (175 ml) almond milk

4 frozen blackberries

1 tablespoon (16 g) peanut butter

2 tablespoons (10 g) protein powder, whey or vegetarian

1 teaspoon Navitas chia seeds (or a comparable brand)

▸ YIELD: SERVES 1

VEGAN BERRY SMOOTHIE

This antioxidant-rich vegan powerhouse has the added benefits of magnesium, omega fatty acids, and protein from the hemp seeds.

1 cup (235 ml) almond milk

4 frozen strawberries

4 frozen raspberries

4 frozen blueberries

1 tablespoon (8 g) Navitas hemp seeds (or a comparable brand)

3 or 4 ice cubes, to taste

▸ YIELD: SERVES 1

CLEANSING GREEN JUICE ▐5▶

This is the perfect elixir to cleanse, restore, and refresh.

½ lemon, juiced

1 small bunch parsley

2 cups (135 g) Tuscan kale, ribs and stems removed

½ cucumber, peeled and coarsely chopped

1 tablespoon (8 g) fresh grated peeled ginger

▸ YIELD: SERVES 1

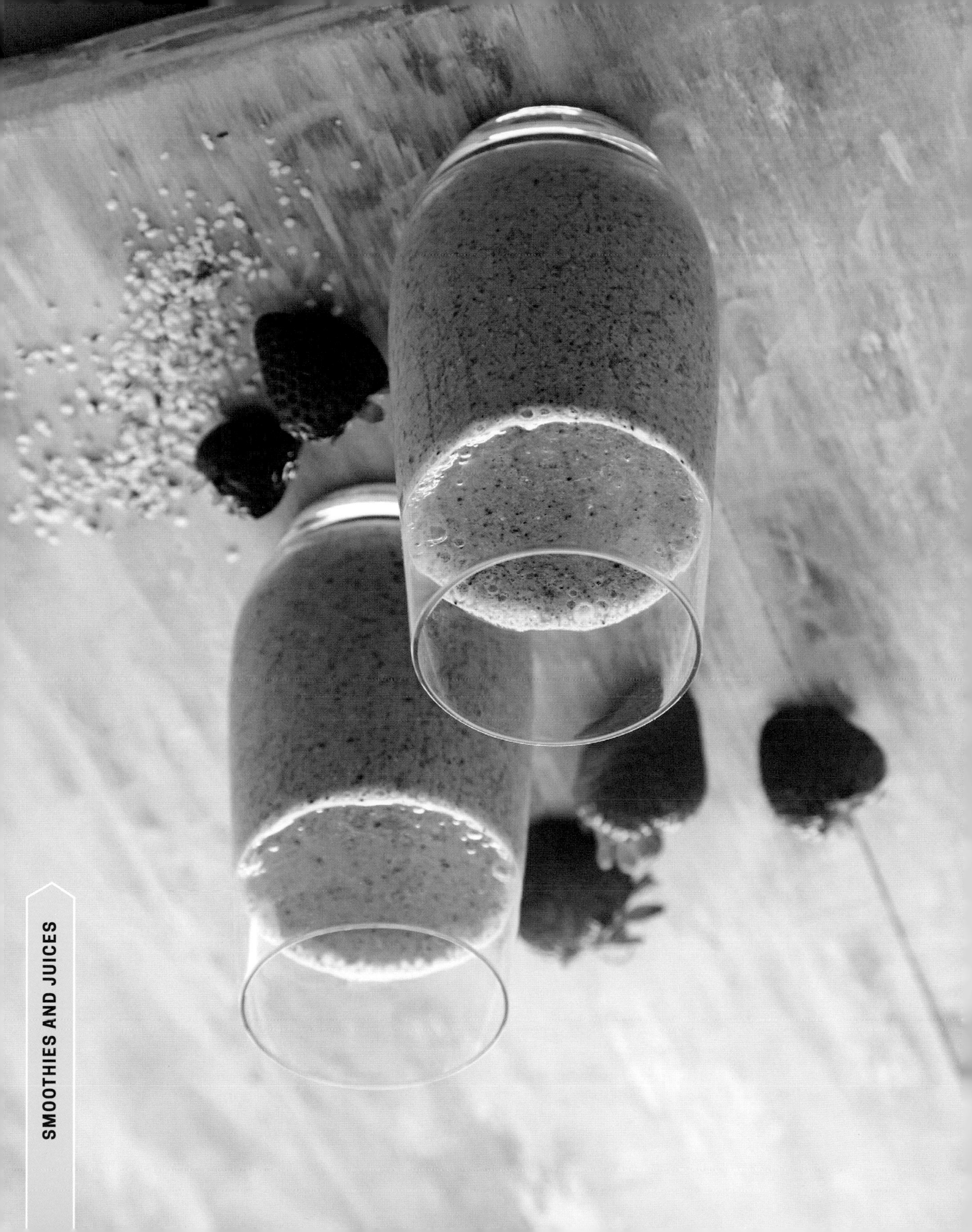

BREAKFAST

The following are just some of the recipes that I have created in my kitchen that I'd like to share with you. Time – or lack thereof – is the most common excuse I hear from my clients for not starting their day with a good, nutritious breakfast. Hopefully, you will find the following nutritious recipes not only tasty, but also easy to prepare and energizing too! Make eating a healthy breakfast a daily ritual!

SPINACH & EGG KIRSCH MUFFINS 15▶

These are tasty little mouthfuls of delicious eggs and spinach made easy with silicon mini-muffin molds.

1 whole egg

2 egg whites

1 teaspoon water

1 teaspoon Dijon mustard

Salt and black pepper, to taste

1 cup (30 g) fresh baby spinach, coarsely chopped

Preheat oven to 350°F (180°C, or gas mark 4).

In a small bowl, gently whisk the whole egg, egg whites, water, mustard, salt, and pepper until well mixed but not too foamy. Set aside.

Wash the spinach leaves and drain but let the spinach stay damp because this water will prevent the spinach from drying out when you cook it. Heat a medium nonstick skillet over high heat and saute the spinach until just wilted.

Place the spinach at the bottom of 10 silicon mini muffin molds. Divide egg white mixture between the molds. Place on a cookie sheet and bake for 8 to 10 minutes or until center is firm to the touch.

▸ **YIELD: 10 MINI MUFFINS, SERVES 2**

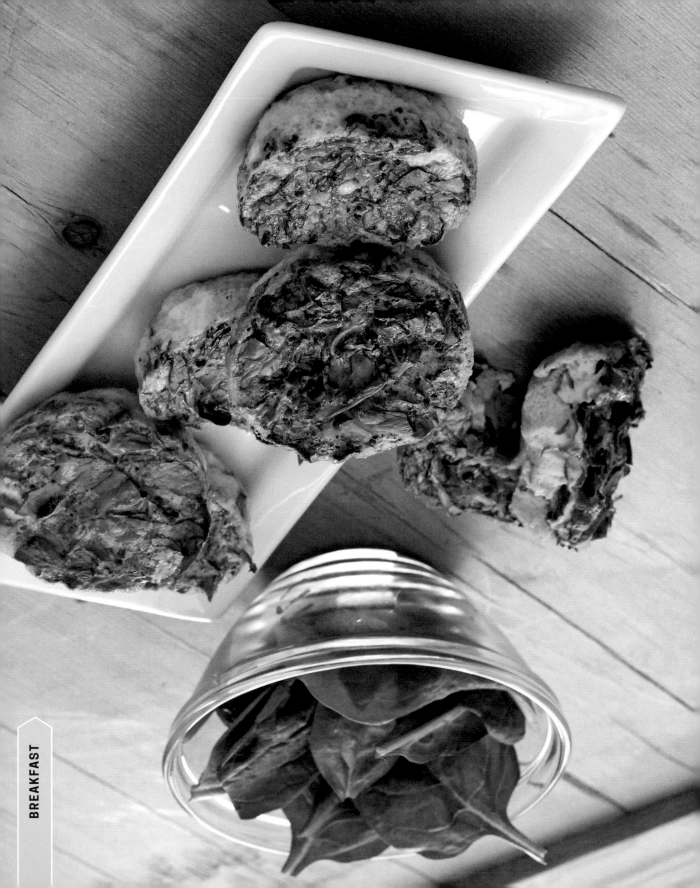

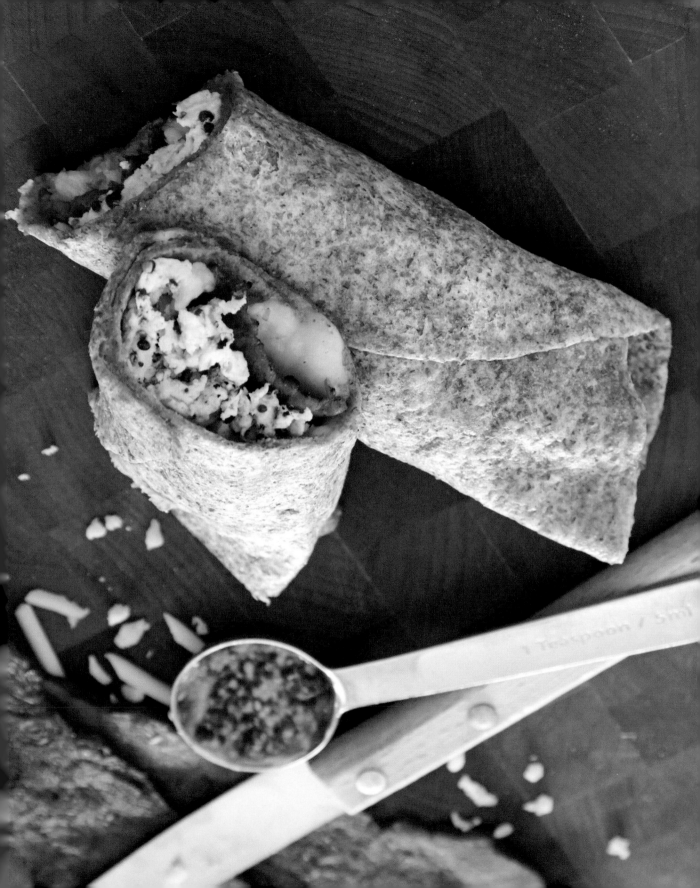

BACON, EGG, AND CHEESE WRAP

This is really a crowd favorite. Who knew that bacon, eggs, and cheese could be so healthy—and tasty, too? It's a great grab-n-go.

1 strip turkey bacon (nitrate-free)

2 large egg whites

1 teaspoon water

1 teaspoon Dijon mustard

Olive oil cooking spray (I use Spectrum Organic brand.)

1 low-carb, high-fiber, whole-wheat wrap

Pepper, to taste

1 slice low-fat Swiss cheese

Preheat oven to 375°F (190°C or gas mark 5).

In a nonstick skillet, cook bacon over medium heat until browned on both sides, about 5 minutes. Remove from pan and blot on paper towel. Set aside.

In a small bowl whisk egg whites, water, and mustard until well blended. Wipe out the skillet and heat over medium heat. Spray with olive oil cooking spray. Cook egg mixture until the egg is just set.

To assemble the wrap, place the wrap on a piece of aluminum foil and top with the egg mixture, turkey bacon, and cheese. Roll and wrap in foil. Place in the oven and cook until the cheese is melted, about 2 minutes. Season with black pepper to taste. Serve warm.

▸ **YIELD: 1 WRAP, SERVES 1**

ROASTED RED PEPPER
KIRSCH EGG MUFFINS [15➤

Add a little vitamin C to your egg muffin.

1 whole large egg

2 egg whites

2 tablespoons (23 g) chopped roasted red bell pepper

1 teaspoon grated Parmesan cheese (This is not allowed on the five-day plan.)

1 tablespoon (4 g) chopped parsley

Pinch cayenne pepper

Salt and black pepper, to taste

Preheat oven to 350°F (180°C, or gas mark 4).

Whisk the whole egg and egg whites in a small bowl. Stir in roasted pepper, Parmesan cheese, and parsley, cayenne pepper, salt, and black pepper. Whisk again until just blended. Spoon mixture into 10 silicon mini muffin molds. Bake for 8 to 10 minutes or until eggs are just set. Serve warm.

▸ **YIELD: 10 MINI MUFFINS, SERVES 2**

THE BEST BERRY YOGURT PARFAIT

This is my go-to breakfast when there is no time to cook. It's the perfect five-minute meal that Emilia and Francesca love to make together.

¾ cup (180 g) plain 2 percent Greek-style yogurt

¾ cup (113 g) mixed berries, gently mashed, with a few whole berries reserved for garnish

1 tablespoon (11 g) chia seeds

¼ cup (4 g) kamut puffs

In a parfait glass or small bowl, layer yogurt, mashed berries, and chia seeds and then top with kamut puffs and sliced whole fruits for garnish.

▸ **YIELD: 1 PARFAIT, SERVES 1**

OATMEAL BANANA BRULEE

Grab a spoonful of potassium with every delicious bite.

1 cup (235 ml) water

½ cup (120 ml) almond milk

½ cup (40 g) uncooked quick steel cut oatmeal

½ teaspoon ground cinnamon

1 banana, peeled and thinly sliced

Bring the water and almond milk to a boil. Add oats and reduce heat to low. Simmer uncovered for 5 minutes.

Stir in cinnamon and continue to cook for 1 minute. Remove from heat and spoon oatmeal into two ovenproof ramekins. Heat the broiler to high. Arrange banana slices over the top of the oatmeal and place under broiler for 3 to 5 minutes until bananas are browned.

▸ **YIELD: SERVES 2**

WHOLE-WHEAT ALMOND PANCAKES

Emilia, Francesca, and I really love to make—and eat—this delicious weekend treat. I serve it with grated apple or berries.

1 cup (125 g) whole-wheat pastry flour

2 teaspoons (9 g) baking powder

⅛ teaspoon ground cinnamon

1 cup (235 ml) unsweetened vanilla almond milk

1 large egg

Coconut oil cooking spray

In a medium bowl mix the flour, baking powder, and cinnamon. Whisk together the almond milk and egg in another small bowl. Pour the almond milk-egg mixture into the dry ingredients and whisk until just blended. Do not overmix.

Heat a nonstick skillet over high heat. Spray with coconut oil spray. Drop ¼ cup (55 g) of batter onto the hot pan and cook until set, about 2 minutes. Turn pancake and continue to cook until lightly browned on both sides. Repeat with remaining batter.

▸ **YIELD: 8 PANCAKES (4 INCHES OR 10-CM EACH), SERVES 2**

Note: Do you want to go gluten-free? Substitute 1 cup (112g) almond flour for the whole-wheat pastry flour.

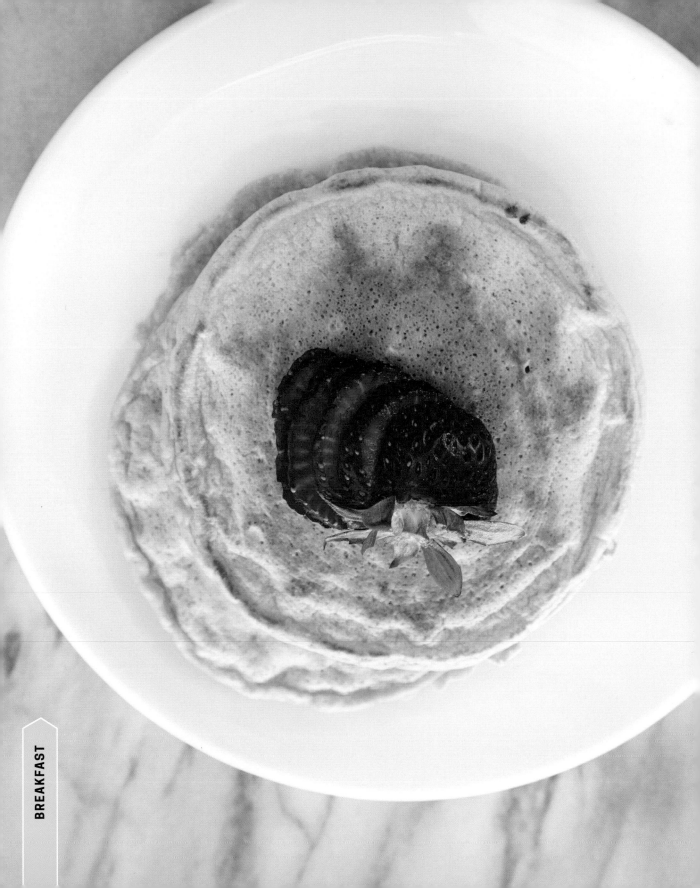

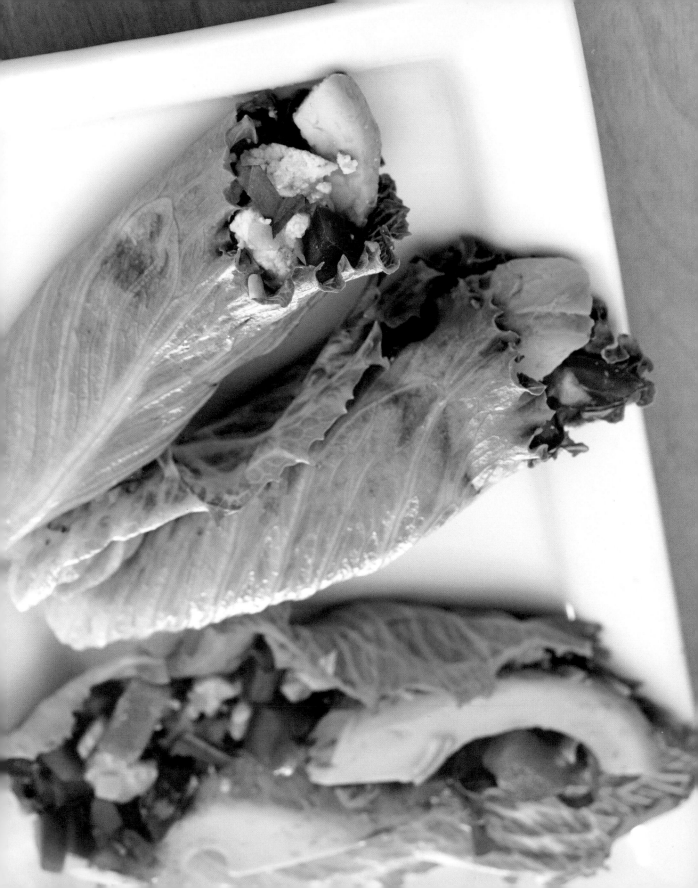

CRUNCHY LETTUCE TOFU TACOS 15▶

To all my vegetarians out there, here is tofu with a Mexican twist. We love it in crunchy lettuce leaves, but it's also perfect in a low-carb, whole-wheat wrap. Enjoy these for breakfast, lunch, or a snack.

Grapeseed oil cooking spray (I use Spectrum Organic brand.)

1 small yellow onion, peeled and chopped

6 ounces (170 g) firm tofu, drained and crumbled

2 tablespoons (30 g) Tomato-Watermelon Salsa (see "Ultimate Family Essentials" section, page 196)

Salt and black pepper, to taste

4 large lettuce leaves, preferably iceberg, washed and dried

½ ripe avocado, peeled and sliced

Spray grapeseed oil cooking spray in a skillet and saute the onions over medium-high heat, stirring to prevent sticking or burning. When the onions start to color, stir in crumbled tofu. Cook for 2 minutes.

Turn off heat, stir in the salsa, and season with salt and black pepper.

Arrange two lettuce leaves on each plate. Divide the tofu mixture on top of the four lettuce leaves and top with sliced avocado. Roll up the lettuce leaves around the mixture.

▶ **YIELD: SERVES 2**

LUNCH

The beauty of the following recipes is that (for the most part) they can be prepared (if not assembled) ahead of time and "brown-bagged." The key to making healthy choices is having them readily available. Whether you're preparing the rice and beans or the quinoa pasta, take the time (15 minutes is all you need) to prepare it in the morning or even the night before. You'll see it's worth the extra effort!

MY BROWN RICE AND BEANS

**I make many versions of this, but this is our new favorite.
It's great as a vegetarian meal or as a little snack.**

Olive oil cooking spray (I use Spectrum Organic brand.)

2 stalks celery, thinly sliced

1 red bell pepper, seeded and coarsely chopped

1 can (15 ounces or 435 g) pinto beans, rinsed and drained

2 cups (330 g) cooked brown rice

¼ cup (40 g) hulled pumpkin seeds

Salt and black pepper, to taste

Spray a pan lightly with olive oil cooking spray and over medium-high heat, saute celery and bell peppers for about 3 minutes. Turn off heat and add beans, rice, and pumpkin seeds and stir to mix. Season with salt and black pepper to taste. Divide into 4 bowls.

▸ **YIELD: SERVES 4**

Note: The rice can be made ahead of time, or you can use boil-in-bag precooked brown rice. Cooking time is 8 to 10 minutes.

GRILLED VEGETABLE WRAP
WITH HUMMUS 15▶

Simple and delicious, this is great for home or a picnic in the park.

Grapeseed oil cooking spray

2 slices summer squash (zucchini or yellow squash)

½ yellow bell pepper, seeded and cut into 2 pieces

Salt and black pepper, to taste

1 tablespoon (15 g) My Ultimate Low-Fat Hummus (See "Ultimate Family Essentials" section, page 198)

1 whole-wheat wrap (This is not allowed on the five-day plan)

½ cucumber peeled, thinly sliced

Heat a grill or grill pan. Wipe grill with grapeseed oil cooking spray. Grill squash and yellow pepper over high heat until vegetables are soft and begin to color. Season with salt and black pepper.

Assemble wrap. Spread hummus down the center of the wrap. Add cucumber, layer with zucchini and peppers, and roll. Cut in half and serve warm.

▸ **YIELD: SERVES 1**

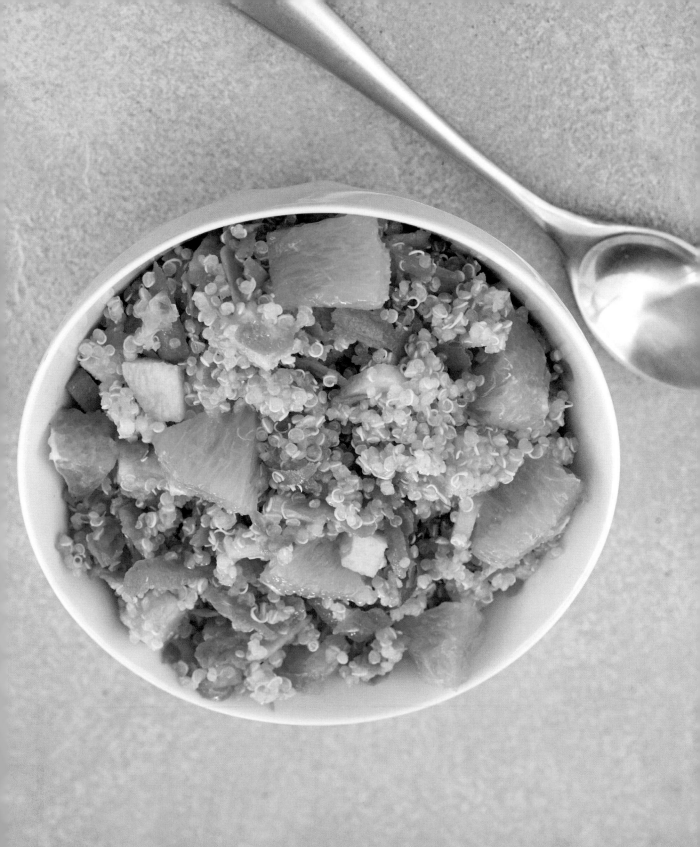

CRUNCHY QUINOA SALAD 15▶

Quinoa is a staple in our kitchen and I've used it in stir-fry, soups, and here in this tasty and satisfying salad.

1 cup (173 g) dried quinoa

1 cup (110 g) coarsely grated peeled carrots

1 cup (130 g) peeled, sliced jicama

2 navel oranges, peeled and sectioned (This is not allowed on the five-day plan.)

2 tablespoons (28 ml) olive oil

Cook the quinoa according to package directions. Meanwhile, prepare the vegetables and oranges.

When the quinoa is cooked, place in a large bowl. Toss gently with the vegetables, oranges, and olive oil. Serve warm or chill for later use.

▸ **YIELD: SERVES 2**

ROASTED TURKEY AVOCADO SALAD

This is the perfect lunch, snack, or teatime treat.

2 cups (68 g) watercress, washed and dried

1 cup (175 g) roasted turkey breast, cubed (See "Ultimate Family Essentials" section, page 198.)

¼ cup (60 g) low-fat (2 percent) Greek yogurt

¼ cup (35 g) toasted pine nuts

Salt and black pepper, to taste

1 ripe avocado, halved and pitted

Coarsely chop 1 cup (34 g) of watercress and place in a small bowl. Stir in turkey breast, yogurt, and pine nuts. Season with salt and black pepper, to taste.

Arrange remaining watercress on two plates. Top with avocado half and fill center of avocado with turkey salad. Place any remaining turkey salad next to the avocado half on the watercress.

▸ **YIELD: SERVES 2**

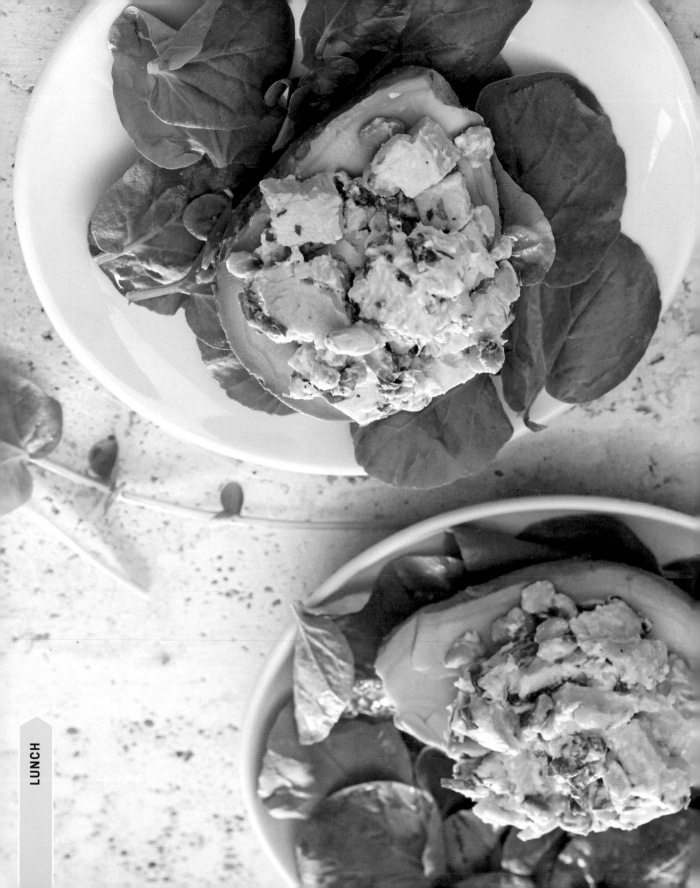

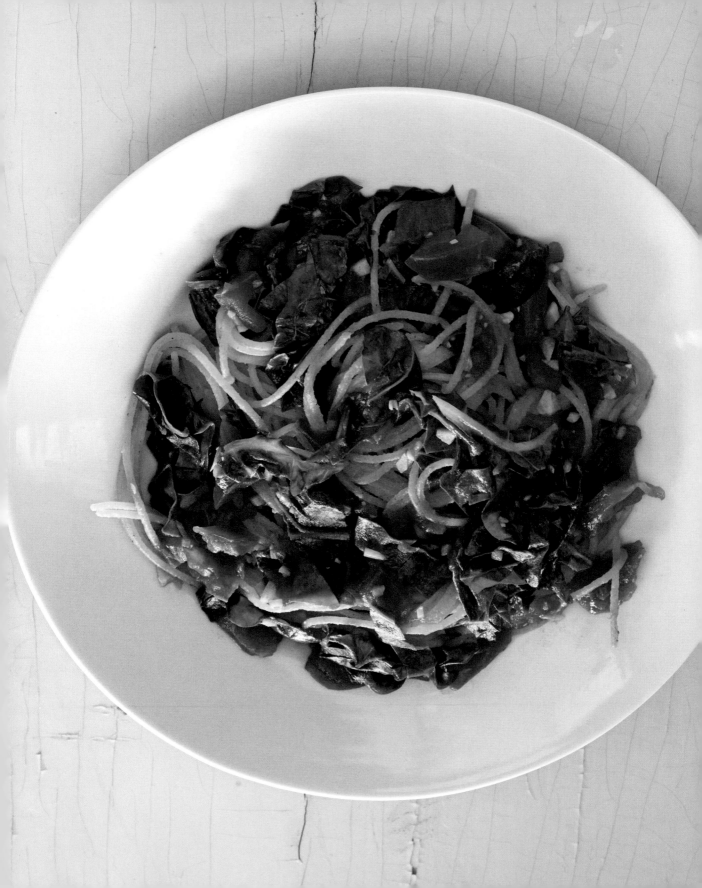

QUINOA SPAGHETTI

What kid doesn't like a warm bowl of pasta? I like the nutty taste of spaghetti made from quinoa and love that it is a source of complete protein. Add the olive oil and tomatoes, and you've got a really healthy meal.

8 ounces (227 g) quinoa spaghetti

2 tablespoons (28 ml) olive oil

3 cloves garlic, minced

1 bunch of Swiss chard, stems and ribs removed, leaves coarsely chopped

1 cup (180 g) chopped tomatoes, either fresh plum tomatoes or canned Italian chopped

Salt and black pepper, to taste

Cook spaghetti according to package instructions.

While pasta cooks, prepare sauce. In a nonstick skillet, heat olive oil and saute garlic over medium heat for 1 minute. Add Swiss chard and continue to cook until wilted. Add chopped tomatoes and cook for 30 seconds more. Season with salt and black pepper and set aside.

Drain cooked spaghetti and return to saucepan. Add sauce to pan and toss to coat spaghetti. Taste and adjust seasonings and then arrange in two bowls.

▸ **YIELD: SERVES 2**

FARRO WITH PARSLEY AND ASPARAGUS

When I was in Italy, I fell in love with farro. This high-fiber, wholesome grain is a great source of iron and protein. I add an egg to make it a complete meal.

1 cup (188 g) uncooked farro

1 cup asparagus cut into 1-inch (2.5-cm) pieces

½ cup (50 g) toasted walnuts, coarsely chopped

4 extra large eggs, poached

¼ cup (15 g) chopped fresh Italian parsley

Salt and pepper, to taste

Cook the farro as directed on the box. While the farro cooks, steam the asparagus until just tender. Drain and place in a medium bowl. Add cooked farro and walnuts, and top with poached egg. Coarsely chop parsley and gently stir into mixture. Season with salt and black pepper to taste.

▸ **YIELD: SERVES 4**

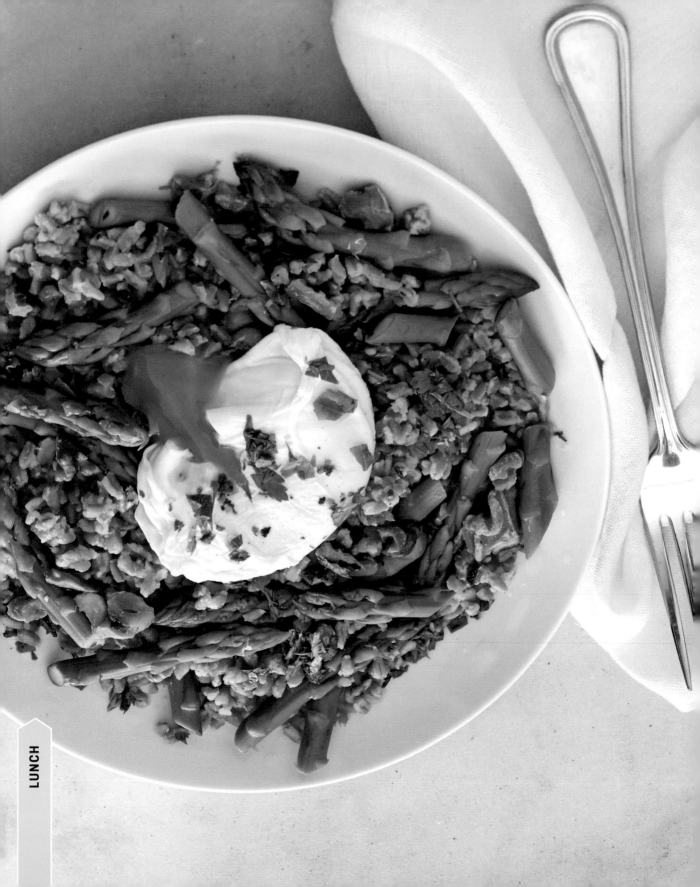

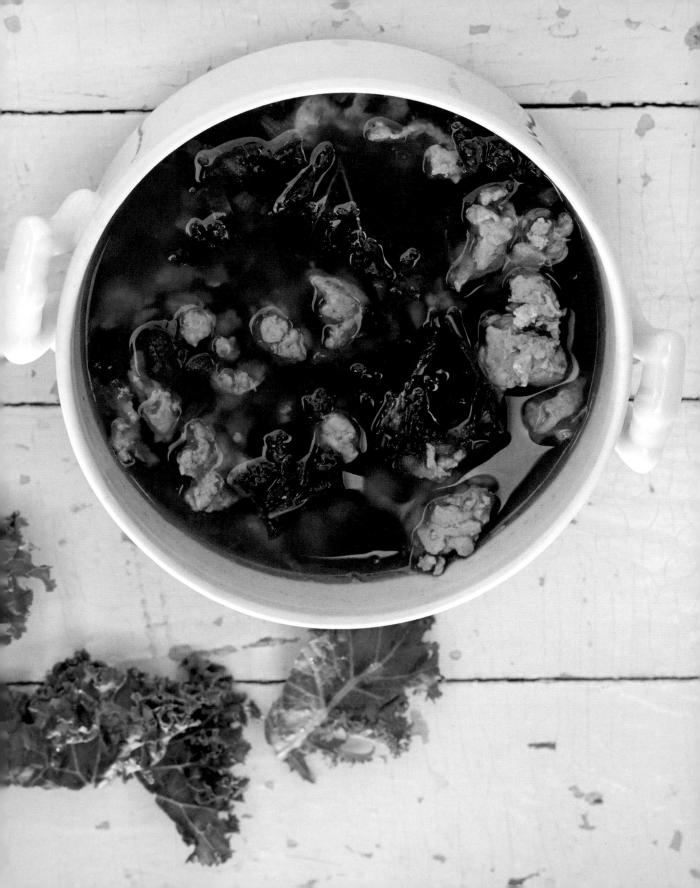

TURKEY KALE SOUP ▐5▶

This soup is a great way to get more of my favorite dark-green vegetable. I love its versatility—it's perfect for lunch, a snack, or dinner.

Grapeseed oil cooking spray

3 shallots, peeled and chopped (about ½ cup [80 g])

¾ pound (340 g) ground turkey, dark meat only

6 cups (1.4 L) Chicken Stock (see "Ultimate Family Essentials" section, page 195.)

1 cup (180 g) diced tomatoes

Salt and black pepper, to taste

2 cups (134 g) trimmed and coarsely chopped kale

Spray a skillet with grapeseed oil cooking spray and saute the shallots over medium heat until they soften but don't brown. Add the ground turkey and brown meat, stirring to break up any big pieces. Add chicken stock and diced tomatoes.

Bring to a boil and season with salt and black pepper to taste. Stir in chopped kale and continue to cook for 1 minute.

▸ **YIELD: SERVES 4**

CHICKEN NOODLE SOUP ▐5▶

Francesca and Emilia's noodle obsession is satisfied with this twist on my grandmother's chicken noodle soup.

6 ounces (171 g) dried soba noodles (This is not allowed on the five-day plan.)

6 cups (1.4 L) Chicken Stock (see "Ultimate Family Essentials" section, page 195.)

Grapeseed oil cooking spray

2 portobello mushroom caps, cubed (about 2 cups [140 g])

8 ounces (226 g) boneless skinless chicken breast, sliced or cubed

2 tablespoons (8 g) chopped fresh parsley

Salt and black pepper, to taste

Oregano, to taste

Cook soba noodles according to package directions. While noodles cook heat chicken broth in another small saucepan.

Heat a nonstick skillet over high heat and spray with grapeseed oil spray. Saute mushrooms until they begin to brown, about 5 minutes. Add chicken and continue to cook over high heat until chicken is cooked through. Season with salt, black pepper, and oregano and set aside.

To serve, arrange the cooked soba noodles and the mushroom-chicken mixture in four bowls and sprinkle chopped parsley over top. Pour warm broth over mixture.

▸ **YIELD: SERVES 4**

DINNER

Since my early childhood, dinner has always been a time to sit down and reflect on the day's events and accomplishments. Complement your day with one of the following delicious and nutritious recipes. Emilia, Francesca, and I would like to share some of our favorite meals. I hope you enjoy them as much as we do!

GRILLED TURKEY BURGERS ▌5▶

There are no dry burgers here. Use moist dark-meat turkey. Serve with Tomato-Watermelon Salsa (see "Ultimate Family Essentials" section, page 196).

1 pound (450 g) skinless turkey thighs, ground (Use breast for the five-day plan.)

½ cup (55 g) coarsely grated carrot

½ cup (53 g) coarsely grated apple (peeled, seeded first)

⅓ cup (27 g) rolled oats

1 tsp (4 g) Dijon mustard

Salt and black pepper, to taste

Grapeseed or olive oil cooking oil or spray

In a medium bowl, combine the ground turkey, carrot, apple, oats, mustard, salt, and black pepper. Use a fork to blend the ingredients until they are evenly incorporated. Divide mixture into four patties.

Heat a cast iron pan (or a grill) over high heat. Rub with grapeseed or olive oil cooking spray or cooking oil. Grill the burgers for about 3 to 4 minutes, then flip. Grill on the other side for another 3 to 4 minutes, or until burger is cooked through.

▸ YIELD: SERVES 4

Note: This very small amount of oats is an exception to the five-day no-grain rule because I love the recipe and it's a negligible amount essential for binding the burger. Plus, oats go a long way in satisfying your appetite. Also, you can purchase ground, skinless, dark meat.

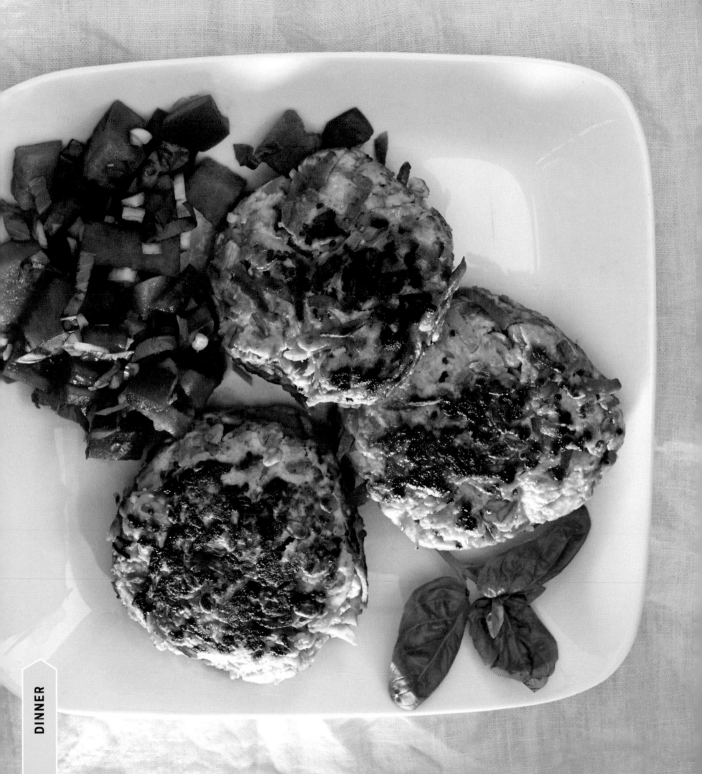

DINNER

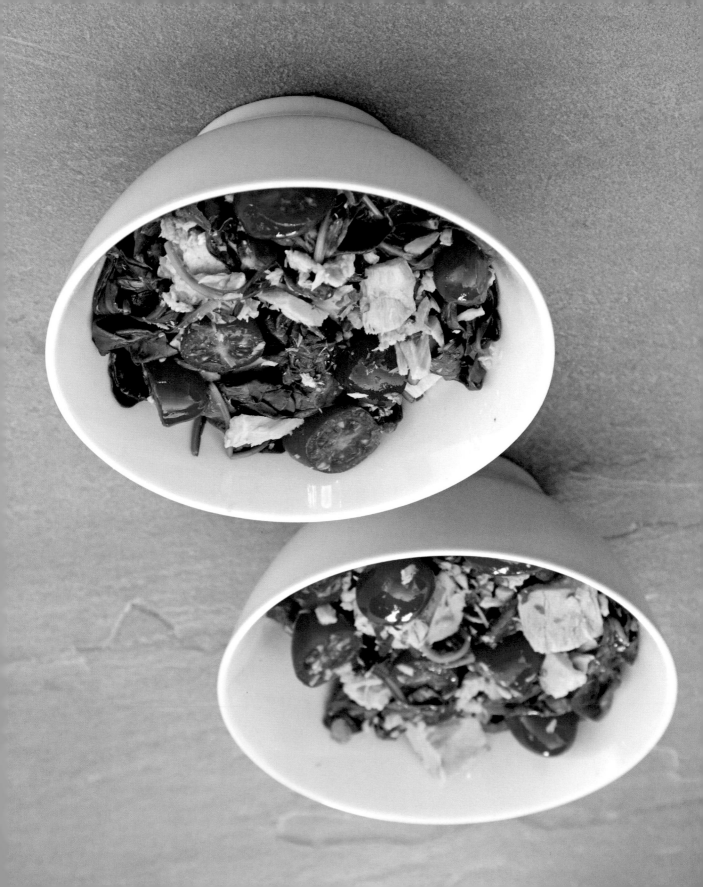

TUNA SPINACH BOWL ▪5▸

Rethink tuna with this five-minute delicious meal.

8 ounces (225 g) baby spinach

1 jar (6.7 ounces [190 g]) Italian tuna

1 cup (150 g) cherry tomatoes, halved

1 ripe avocado, peeled, pitted, and cubed

¼ cup (36 g) toasted almonds, coarsely chopped

Salt and black pepper, to taste

Wash the spinach and while still damp place in a pan over medium heat until just wilted. Turn off the heat and toss remaining ingredients into saute pan. Mix everything together and serve.

▸ **YIELD: SERVES 2**

CHICKEN CASHEW STIR-FRY ▶5

This is delicious, nutritious, and oh-so-easy to prepare.

8 ounces (226 g) boneless skinless chicken breast cut into 1-inch (2.5-cm) strips

Almond-Lime Marinade (See "Ultimate Family Essentials" section, page 196)

Grapeseed oil cooking spray

2 cloves garlic, minced

1 red bell pepper, seeded and cut into thin strips

½ cup (68 g) raw cashews

▶ **YIELD: SERVES 2**

In a small bowl, mix the chicken with the Almond-Lime Marinade to coat evenly. Cover and let sit at room temperature for 5 minutes or refrigerate for up to 8 hours.

Heat a cast iron skillet over high heat and spray with grapeseed oil cooking spray. Add garlic, red peppers, and cashews and cook for 1 minute until garlic and cashews begin to brown slightly. Add marinated chicken and cook until chicken is cooked through, about 5 minutes.

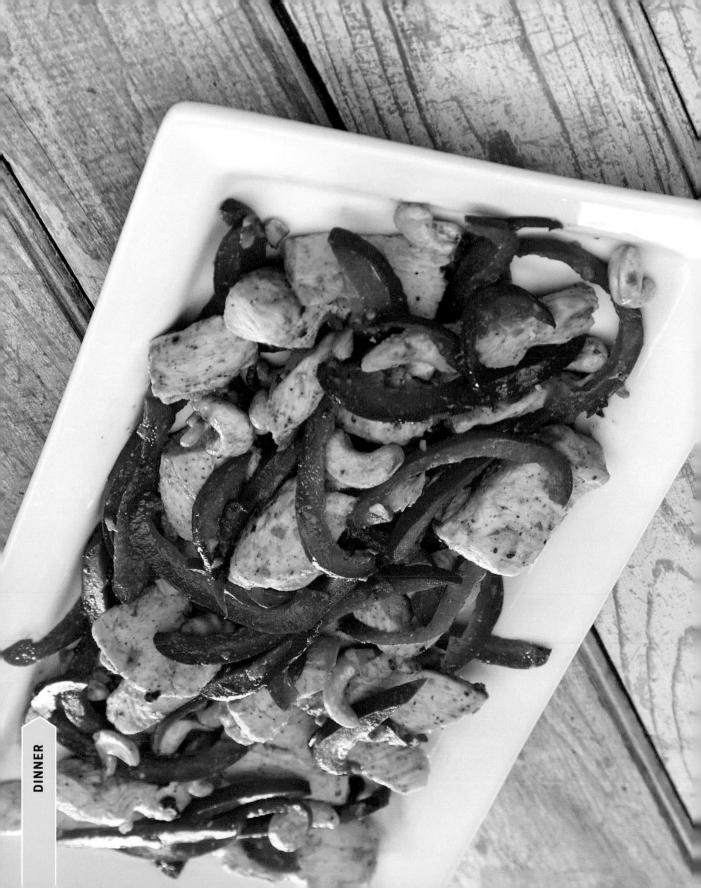

DINNER

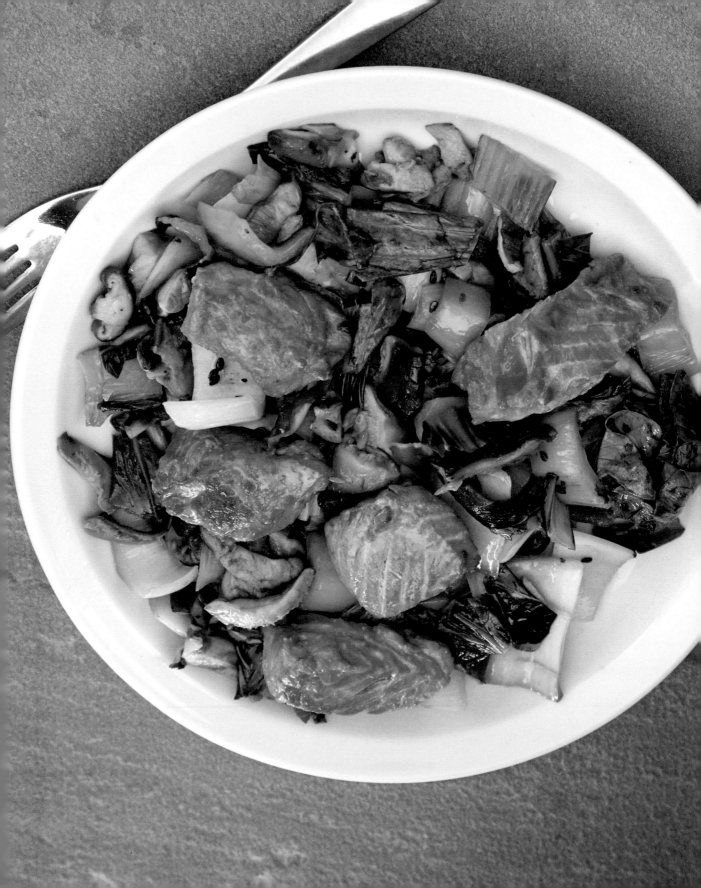

CRISPY SALMON NUGGETS ▪5▶

Bite-sized pieces of salmon are the perfect excuse for Emilia and Francesca to gobble these up with their hands.

8 ounces (226 g) wild salmon filet, skin removed

3 tablespoons (24 g) grated fresh ginger

2 tablespoons (28 ml) lemon juice

2 tablespoons (28 ml) low-sodium tamari sauce

1 tablespoon (15 ml) grapeseed oil, plus more for cooking

Cut salmon into 2-inch (5 cm) cubes. In a medium bowl, whisk together ginger, lemon juice, tamari sauce, and 1 tablespoon (15 ml) grapeseed oil. Add salmon cubes. Toss gently to coat and set aside for 5 minutes.

Heat a cast iron skillet over high heat. Rub or spray with grapeseed oil as needed. Cook the salmon cubes over high heat until cooked through, about 2 minutes on each side.

▸ **YIELD: SERVES 2**

Note: I like to serve this with Bok Choy with Maitake Mushrooms, page 188.

THAI GINGER SIRLOIN SALAD

This is a simplified version of one of the more popular dishes from my first book, *Sound Mind, Sound Body*.

8 ounces (227 g) sirloin steak, trimmed of fat

Ginger-Soy Dressing (See "Ultimate Family Essentials" section, page 194.)

2 cups (110 g) mesclun greens (or salad greens of your choice), washed and dried

Grapeseed oil cooking spray

1 cup (65 g) sugar snaps, trimmed and cut on bias into quarters

½ cup (55 g) grated carrots

1 teaspoon toasted sesame seeds

Cut the sirloin into ½-inch (1.3-cm) slices and place in a small bowl with the Ginger-Soy Dressing. Marinate at room temperature for 5 minutes.

While the meat marinates, arrange mixed greens and grated carrots on two plates.

Heat a cast iron skillet over medium heat and spray with grapeseed oil cooking spray. Add the sugar snap peas and cook until bright green and still crunchy, about 1 to 2 minutes. Remove from heat and arrange sugar snaps on the lettuce.

In that same pan, sear sirloin slices for 30 seconds on each side. Add Ginger-Soy Dressing to pan and bring to a boil. Remove from heat immediately and arrange steak slices on the two plates. Drizzle with pan juices and sprinkle with toasted sesame seeds.

▸ **YIELD: SERVES 2**

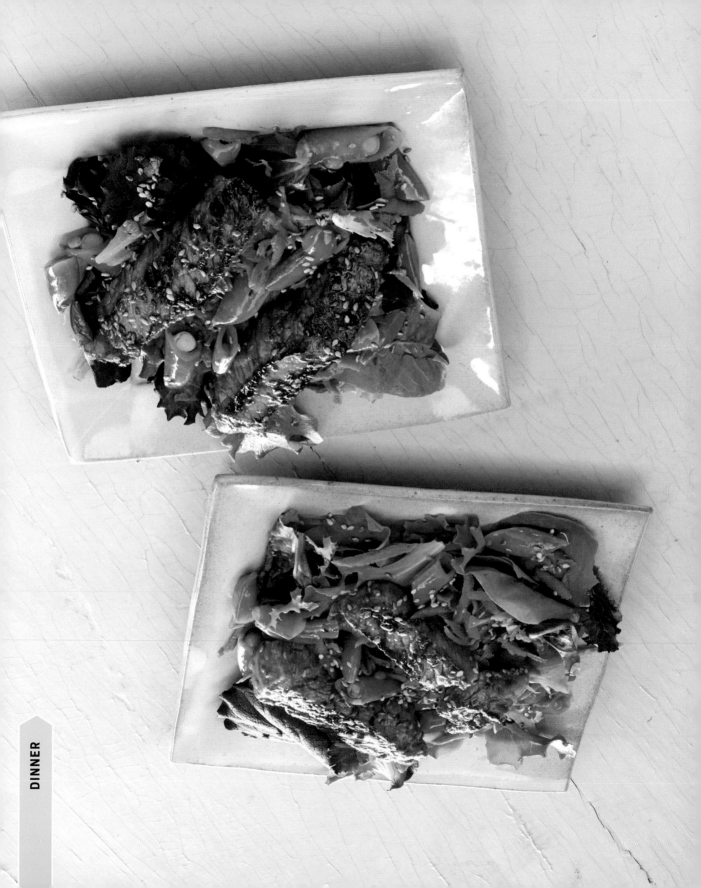

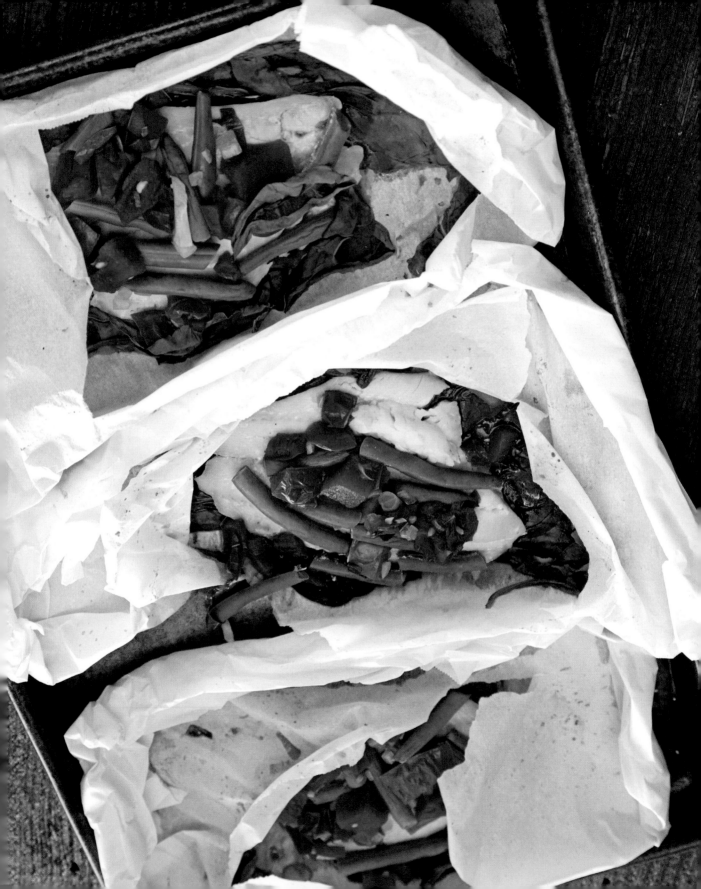

STEAMED FISH IN PARCHMENT ▌5▶

**This recipe takes a little work to assemble, but the end result is worth the effort.
Serve each parchment packet on a plate for your guests to open.**

**4 wild sole or flounder fillets
(6 ounces [170 g] each)**

4 cups (120 g) baby spinach

**½ pound (150 g) string beans, ends
trimmed and cut into 2-inch (5 cm)
pieces**

**Tomato-Watermelon Salsa (See
"Ultimate Family Essentials"
section, page 196.)**

1 tablespoon (15 ml) olive oil

Salt and black pepper, to taste

**4 pieces (13 x 13 inch [33 x 33 cm])
parchment paper**

Preheat oven to 375°F (190°C, or gas mark 5).

Arrange the parchment paper on a large work surface. Place 1 cup (40 g) of spinach in the center of each paper. Lay one fish filet on top of the spinach. Season with salt and black pepper.

Top each filet with ¼ of the string beans and salsa. Drizzle with olive oil. Fold parchment over fish and place on baking sheet. Bake for 8 to 10 minutes until fish is cooked through. Place parchment packets on plates and serve.

▸ **YIELD: SERVES 4**

SAUTEED COLLARD GREENS WITH LENTILS 15▶

This is a nutrient-rich vegan dinner.

Grapeseed oil cooking spray

4 cups (144 g) coarsely chopped collard greens

1 medium onion, peeled and thinly sliced

½ sweet bell pepper, seeded and thinly sliced

½ teaspoon ground turmeric

1 cup (192 g) cooked lentils

Salt and black pepper, to taste

Wash and trim collard greens, then coarsely chop.

Heat a pan over high heat. Spray with grapeseed oil cooking spray. Add onion and pepper and saute until wilted and onion just begins to color, about 4 minutes. Add turmeric and stir to coat.

Add collard greens and continue to cook until wilted, about 1 minute. Stir in lentils and season with salt and black pepper to taste.

▶ YIELD: SERVES 2

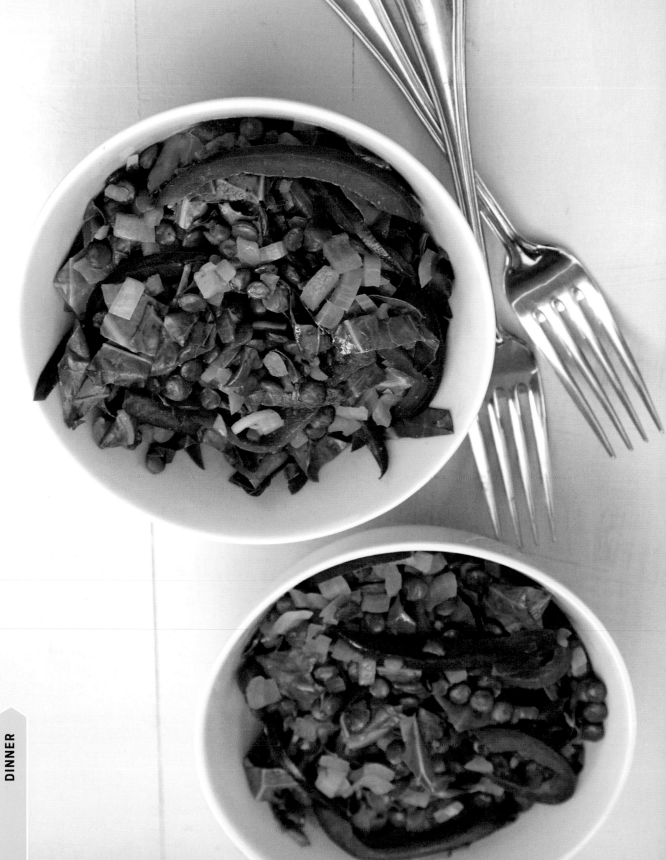

SIDES

Never one to miss an opportunity to add some more nutrients to your meal, the following sides do just that in an easy-to-prepare, tasty way.

CRUNCHY ROMAINE AVOCADO SALAD [5▶

This is my version of a Waldorf salad. I use crunchy shredded romaine lettuce and substitute avocado for the traditional celery. Sometimes I top this with grilled chicken for lunch.

1 small head romaine lettuce, washed and shredded (about 4 cups [220 g])

1 apple, washed, cored, and thinly sliced (This is not allowed on the five-day plan.)

¼ cup (30 g) toasted, coarsely chopped walnuts

1 ripe avocado, peeled, pitted, and cubed

Apple Cider Vinaigrette (See "Ultimate Family Essentials" section, page 194.)

In a large bowl, toss all ingredients together and serve.

▸ YIELD: SERVES 4

KALE SALAD 15▶

I found and adapted this Thanksgiving staple from *Bon Appetit* magazine a few years ago. It is so delicious.

2 cups (134 g) shredded kale

1½ cups (132 g) shredded Brussels sprouts

Meyer Lemon Vinaigrette (See "Ultimate Family Essentials" section, page 195.)

⅓ cup (33 g) grated pecorino (This is not allowed on the five-day plan.)

¼ cup (28 g) toasted, coarsely

chopped peeled hazelnuts

In a medium bowl mix together kale, Brussels sprouts, and Meyer Lemon Vinaigrette. Toss salad with your hands to coat vegetables with the dressing. Gently stir in cheese and hazelnuts.

▶ **YIELD: SERVES 2**

CAULIFLOWER MASH 15▶

It looks and feels like mashed potatoes, but it's healthier.

1 head of cauliflower, washed, trimmed, and broken into florets

1 tablespoon (15 ml) olive oil

2 cloves garlic, peeled and thinly sliced

1 cup (70 g) sliced shiitake mushrooms

¼ cup (60 ml) Chicken Stock (See "Ultimate Family Essentials" section, page TK.)

Set a large saucepan with water to boil over high heat. Cook cauliflower florets in boiling water for 5 to 7 minutes until tender.

While cauliflower cooks heat oil in a nonstick skillet over high heat. Saute garlic for 1 minute and add mushrooms. Continue to cook until mushrooms and garlic are lightly browned. Set aside.

Drain and puree cooked cauliflower in a food processor or blender with Chicken Stock until smooth. Season with salt and pepper, to taste.

Spoon into a serving bowl and top with sauteed mushrooms.

▶ **YIELD: SERVES 4**

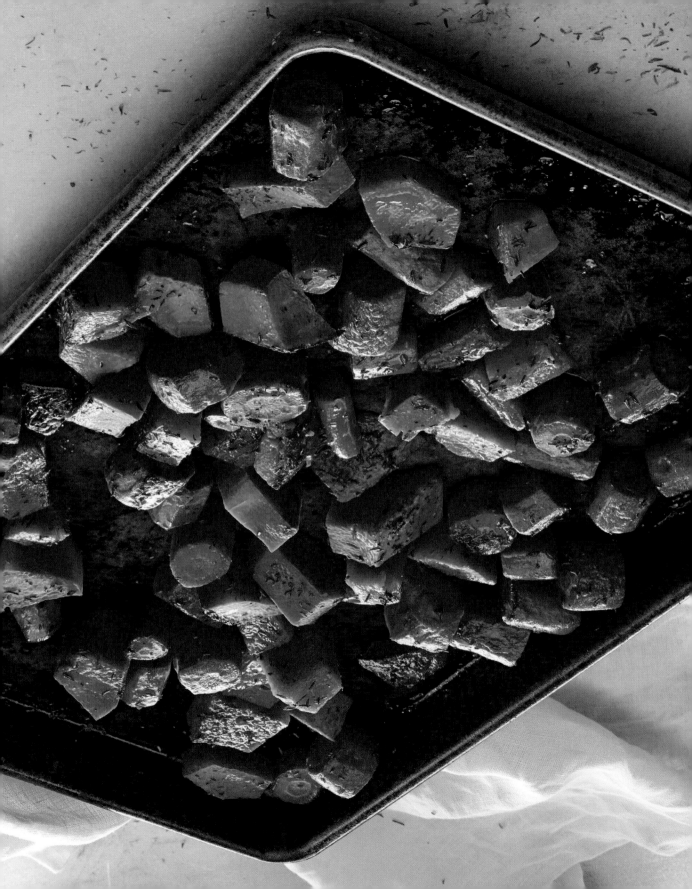

ROASTED CARROTS AND SQUASH WITH FRESH THYME

I love to use carrots and sweet butternut squash, but other vegetables such as Brussels sprouts, cauliflower, fennel, and acorn squash all roast beautifully using this technique. A quick blanching and a very hot oven cut roasting times in half.

1 cup (130 g) peeled, sliced carrots, cut into 1-inch (2.5 cm) slices

1 cup (140 g) peeled, butternut squash, cut into 1-inch (2.5 cm) cubes

½ teaspoon dried thyme

¼ teaspoon kosher salt

1 tablespoon (15 ml) olive oil

Preheat oven to 500°F (250°C, or gas mark 10).

Place vegetables in small pot of briskly boiling water. Return to a boil and continue to cook for 3 minutes. Drain vegetables and toss immediately with thyme leaves, salt, and olive oil.

Roast in a small roasting pan for 8 to 10 minutes until vegetables are lightly browned.

▶ YIELD: SERVES 2

BOK CHOY WITH MAITAKE MUSHROOMS 15▶

I like to use maitake (also known as hen-of-the-wood) mushrooms to make this delicious, crunchy side dish. Prized in Japanese and Chinese cooking for their taste and immune-boosting properties, maitake are gaining popularity in the United States. If you can't find these mushrooms, use shitake or oyster mushrooms instead.

Olive oil cooking spray (I use Spectrum brand.)

3 cups (210 g) baby bok choy, coarsely chopped

1 cup (70 g) sliced maitake mushrooms

3 cloves garlic, minced

1 tablespoon (8 g) black sesame seeds

1 teaspoon toasted sesame oil

Salt and black pepper, to taste

Heat a pan over medium heat and spray with olive oil cooking spray. Saute garlic until it just begins to color lightly, about 1 minute.

Add mushrooms and bok choy and saute over high heat for 3 to 4 minutes until vegetables are cooked but still crispy. Stir in sesame seeds and continue to cook for 1 minute. Turn off heat and stir in sesame oil. Add salt and black pepper to taste.

▶ **YIELD: SERVES 2**

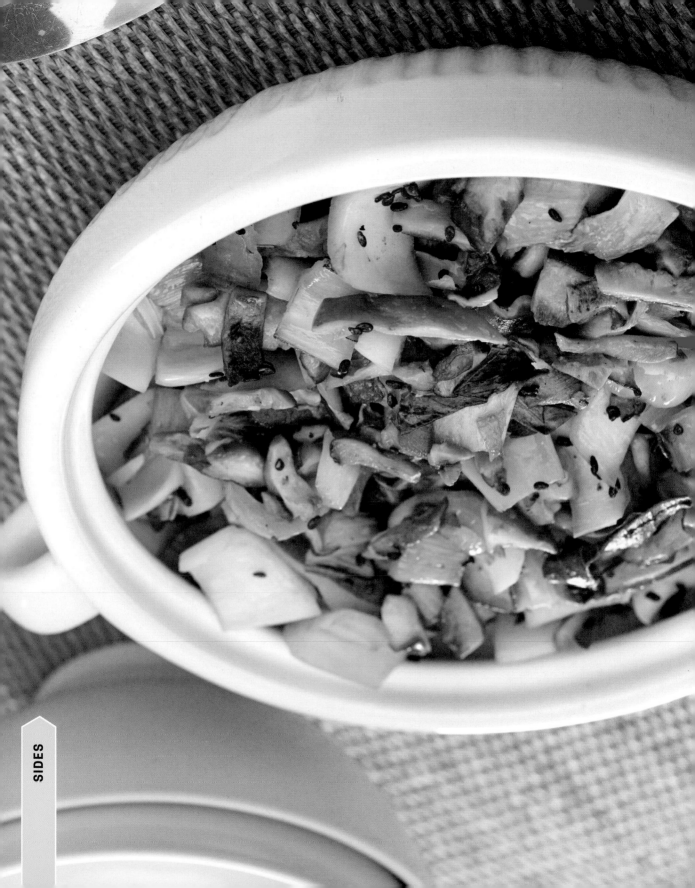

SIDES

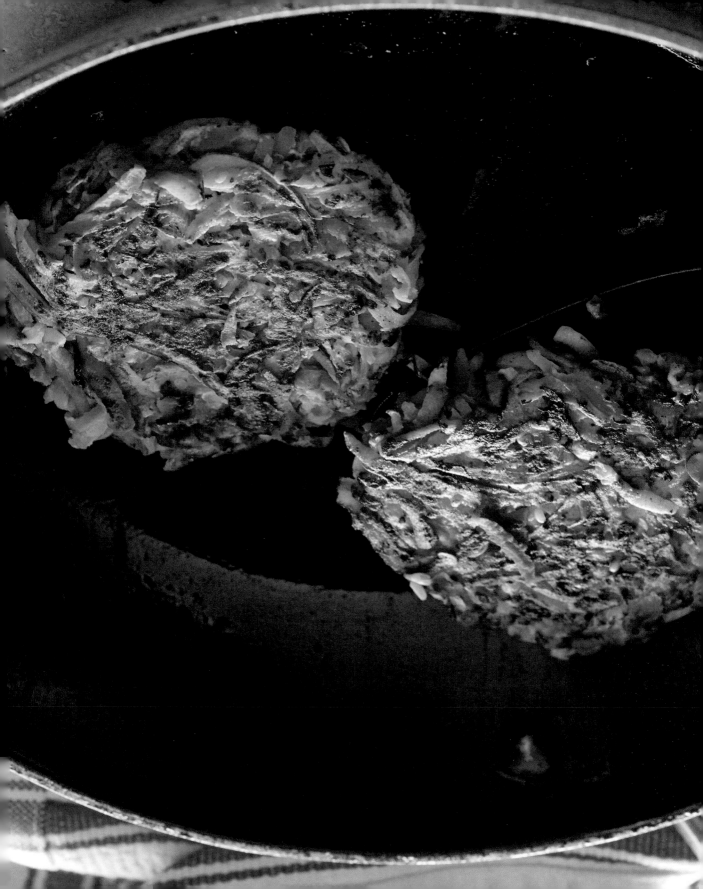

ZUCCHINI SCALLION PANCAKES

Emilia and Francesca really love these pancakes. They are sinfully good as a snack or even as a side with one of the lunch salads such as the Crunchy Romaine Avocado Salad on page 184.

1 cup (120 g) coarsely grated zucchini

¾ cup (100 g) finely grated sweet potato

¼ cup (25 g) chopped scallions

2 tablespoons (14 g) flax meal (ground flaxseeds)

1 egg

Salt and black pepper to taste

Grapeseed or Olive oil cooking spray

Mix all ingredients (through salt and pepper) in a medium bowl. Shape mixture into four 4-inch (10 cm) pancakes.

Heat a nonstick skillet over medium heat. Spray with grapeseed or olive oil cooking spray. Cook pancakes for 5 minutes on each side until browned.

▸ **YIELD: SERVES 4**

CRUNCHY STIR-FRY 15▶

This side is a cross between a stir-fry and a slaw. I like my cauliflower and broccoli cooked a little but still crunchy. Add some Napa cabbage and Ginger-Soy Dressing (found on page 194) and you will never go back to traditional coleslaw.

Olive oil cooking spray (I use Spectrum brand.)

½ cup (80 g) chopped onion

1 cup (71 g) broccoli florets cut into bite-sized pieces

1 cup (132 g) cauliflower florets cut into bite-sized pieces

1½ cups (105 g) shredded Napa cabbage

Ginger-Soy Dressing (See "Ultimate Family Essentials" section, page 194.)

Spray a pan with olive oil cooking spray. Heat over medium heat. Add onions and cook for 2 to 3 minutes, stirring frequently to prevent sticking.

Raise heat to high and add broccoli and cauliflower florets. Cook until vegetables begin to brown but are still crunchy, about 4 minutes. Remove from heat and stir in Napa cabbage and Ginger-Soy Dressing.

▸ **YIELD: SERVES 2**

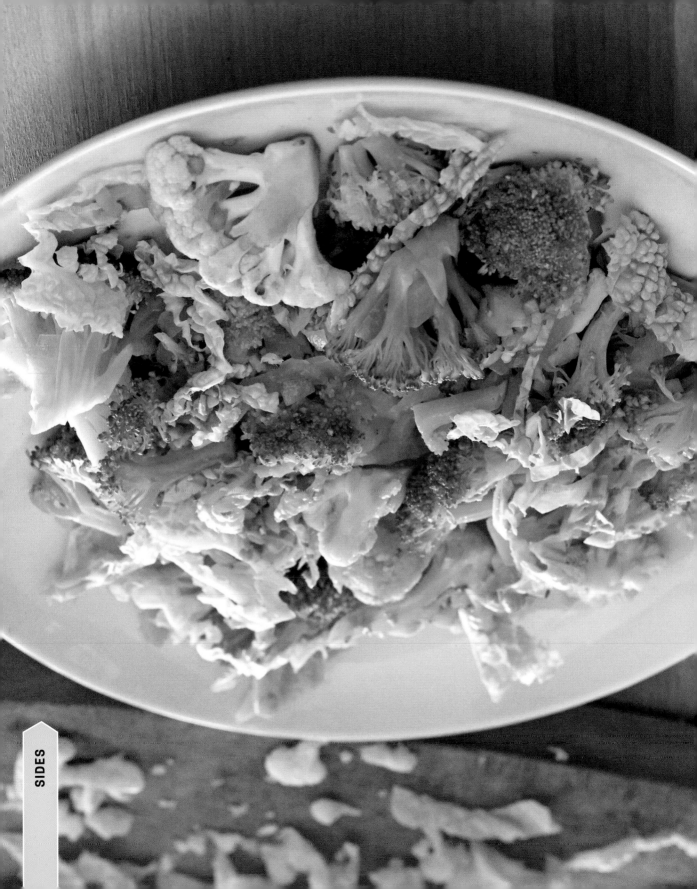

ULTIMATE FAMILY ESSENTIALS

Turkey breast, hummus, and salsa are a few of my go-to snacks and meal staples. I like to keep them, along with my favorite dressings, salsa, stock, and marinade, readily available. Like all of my recipes, these are short on preparation time and long on flavor!

APPLE CIDER VINAIGRETTE

A light, refreshing dressing, I like to add to my Crunchy Romaine Avocado Salad, page 184.

2 tablespoons (28 ml) apple cider vinegar

1 tablespoon (15 ml) olive oil

2 tablespoons (30 g) low-fat (2 percent) Greek yogurt

1 tablespoon (10 g) chopped shallots

Salt and black pepper, to taste

Whisk together all ingredients in a small bowl.

▸ **YIELD: SERVES 2**

GINGER-SOY DRESSING ◼5▶

This is a tasty, versatile dressing that I like to use with roasted chicken and fish.

1 tablespoon (15 ml) organic low-sodium tamari or soy sauce

2 tablespoons (28 ml) rice wine vinegar

2 teaspoons (10 ml) sesame oil

2 teaspoons (5 g) finely grated fresh ginger root

1 tablespoon (8 g) toasted sesame seeds

Mix together all ingredients in a small bowl.

▸ **YIELD: SERVES 2**

STRAWBERRY VINAIGRETTE

Add a little fruity flavor and vitamin C to your dressing.

1/4 cup (60 ml) red wine vinegar

2 tablespoons (28 ml) bottled water

1 tablespoon (15 ml) lemon juice

1 tablespoon (11 g) Dijon mustard

2 frozen strawberries + 1 tablespoon (15 ml) of bottled water

Fresh ground black pepper

In a small bowl or glass jar, combine the vinegar, water, lemon juice, and mustard and set aside. Puree two frozen strawberries and 1 tablespoon of water. Add the strawberry mixture to the vinaigrette and whisk until mixed. Use immediately or store in the refrigerator for up to one week.

▸ YIELD: SERVES 2

CHICKEN STOCK ▐5▶

I always have plenty of this in the fridge and backup in the freezer.

1 whole, bone-in chicken (about 3 pounds [1.5 kg])

4 quarts (3.8 L) cold bottled water

1 vidalia onion, chopped

2 celery ribs, greens included, chopped

2 spring onions or scallions, chopped

1 garlic clove, minced

1 bunch parsley

4 to 5 sprigs fresh thyme or 1 teaspoon dried

1 tablespoon (5 g) tricolored peppercorns or 2 teaspoons (4 g) fresh coarsely ground black pepper

1 bay leaf

Wash and cut the chicken into pieces at the joints (or have your butcher do it). Place the chicken in a large stockpot. Add the water and bring to a boil over high heat. Skim any foam that rises to the surface. Add the onion, celery, spring onions/scallions, and garlic. Return to a boil and then immediately reduce the heat to medium-low. Gently simmer for 2 hours, uncovered, skimming the foam occasionally and adding more water if necessary to keep the chicken submerged.

Add the parsley, thyme, peppercorns/black pepper, and bay leaf. Simmer for 1 hour more.

Strain the stock through a sieve, pressing the solids to extract the liquid. Discard the solids. Pull the chicken meat off the bones and reserve for another use. Let the stock cool to room temperature and then refrigerate until cold. Remove and discard the fat that congeals on the surface. Pour the stock into ice cube trays and freeze until solid. Transfer the cubes to freezer bags and freeze for up to three months.

▸ YIELD: 2 QUARTS (1.9 L)

TOMATO-WATERMELON SALSA

This treat brings me back to summer, even on the coldest days of winter.

1½ cups (270 g) cubed ripe tomatoes

½ cup (75 g) cubed seedless watermelon

1 shallot, peeled and minced

2 tablespoons (28 ml) fresh lime juice

¼ cup (10 g) basil leaves, washed and julienned

Salt and black pepper, to taste

Mix all ingredients together in a medium bowl. Serve immediately.

▸ **YIELD: SERVES 4**

Note: If you like a little bit of heat, stir in one seeded and chopped jalapeño pepper.

ALMOND-LIME MARINADE ◼5▸

This is a versatile marinade that I use in my Chicken Cashew Stir-Fry (page 174), but it's great to marinate any poultry or seafood or to tenderize meat.

1 lime, juiced

1 tablespoon (15 ml) water

1 tablespoon (16 g) almond butter

Dash cayenne pepper

Dash turmeric

Pinch black pepper

Pinch salt

In a small bowl, whisk together all ingredients.

▸ **YIELD: SERVES 2**

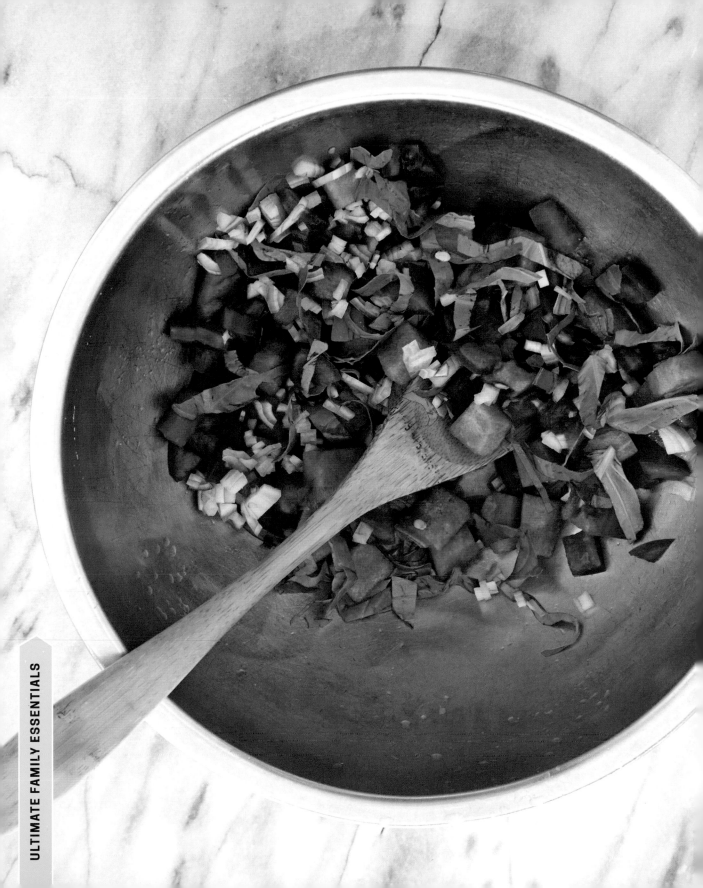

ROASTED ROSEMARY SAGE TURKEY BREAST ▌5▶

Emilia, Francesca, and I really love turkey breast so many different ways—as a snack with carrots and celery sticks after lunch or served in an avocado as turkey salad. I make a breast on the weekend and enjoy it for the week.

1 whole turkey breast (about 3 to 5 pounds [1.4 to 1.8 kg])

1 lemon, halved

1 small bunch fresh sage

3 sprigs fresh rosemary

1 tablespoon (15 ml) olive oil

Salt and black pepper, to taste

Preheat oven to 350°F (180°C, or gas mark 4).

Rinse turkey breast and pat dry. Place lemon and herbs in turkey cavity. Rub olive oil over turkey breast and season with salt and black pepper.

Bake for about 1½ hours until a meat thermometer registers 170°F (77°C). Remove from oven and let rest at least 15 minutes before slicing.

▸ **YIELD: 3 TO 5 POUNDS**

MY ULTIMATE LOW-FAT HUMMUS

This is a very versatile staple in my pantry. I use it in my vegetable wrap for lunch. It is also the perfect snack, as I like to pair it in a roasted turkey cucumber roll-up. Use it as is or turn up the heat with extra cayenne pepper or a chopped jalapeño.

1½ cups (360 g) cooked or canned chickpeas, rinsed and drained

¼ cup (60 g) 2 percent Greek style yogurt

1 clove garlic, minced

1 lemon, juiced

Salt and black pepper, to taste

Cayenne pepper (optional)

1 tablespoon (4 g) chopped parsley

In a food processor, combine the chickpeas, yogurt, garlic, and lemon juice. Process until smooth. Season to taste with salt, black pepper, and cayenne pepper if desired. Stir in parsley and serve.

▸ **YIELD: SERVES 4**

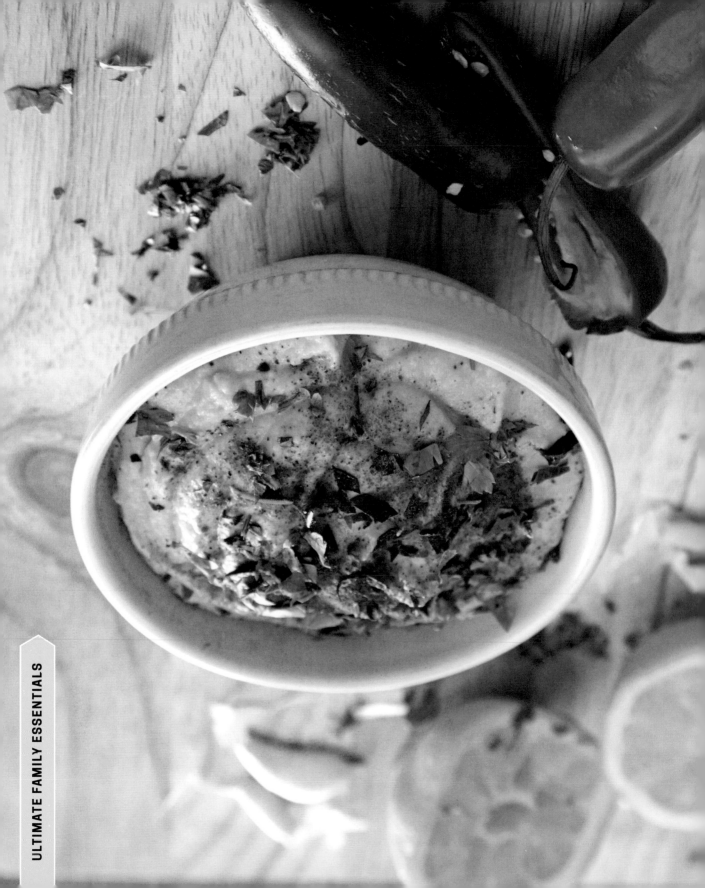

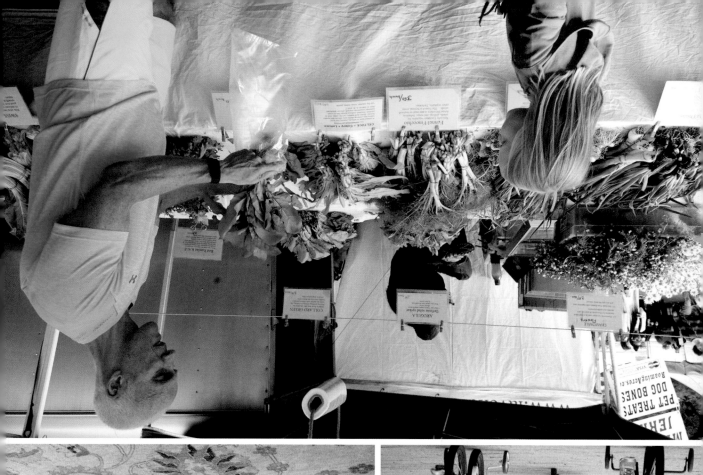
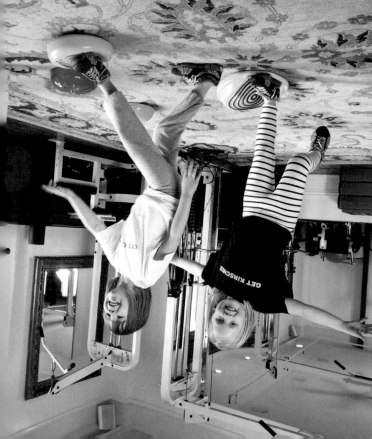
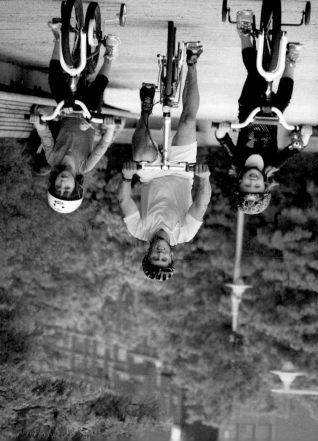

MANAGEMENT AND MAINTENANCE MADE EASY

Chapter 5

MANAGING THE FIVE-DAY PLAN

The trackers in the first half of this chapter will give you everything you
need to know and do for the 5-5-5 Program's super powerful five-day plan
to five pounds of weight loss.

Five-Day Exercise Tracker

Here is your five-day menu of exercises arranged
by body type. Each exercise is explained step by
step in chapter 2. Be sure you brush up on each
movement before you begin your five minutes
of exercise because keeping up the intensity and
sticking to the prescribed timing are keys
to success.

If you are doing more than one five-minute
session per day, you can repeat the same circuit
throughout the day or mix it up using exercises
listed for other days or even other body types.

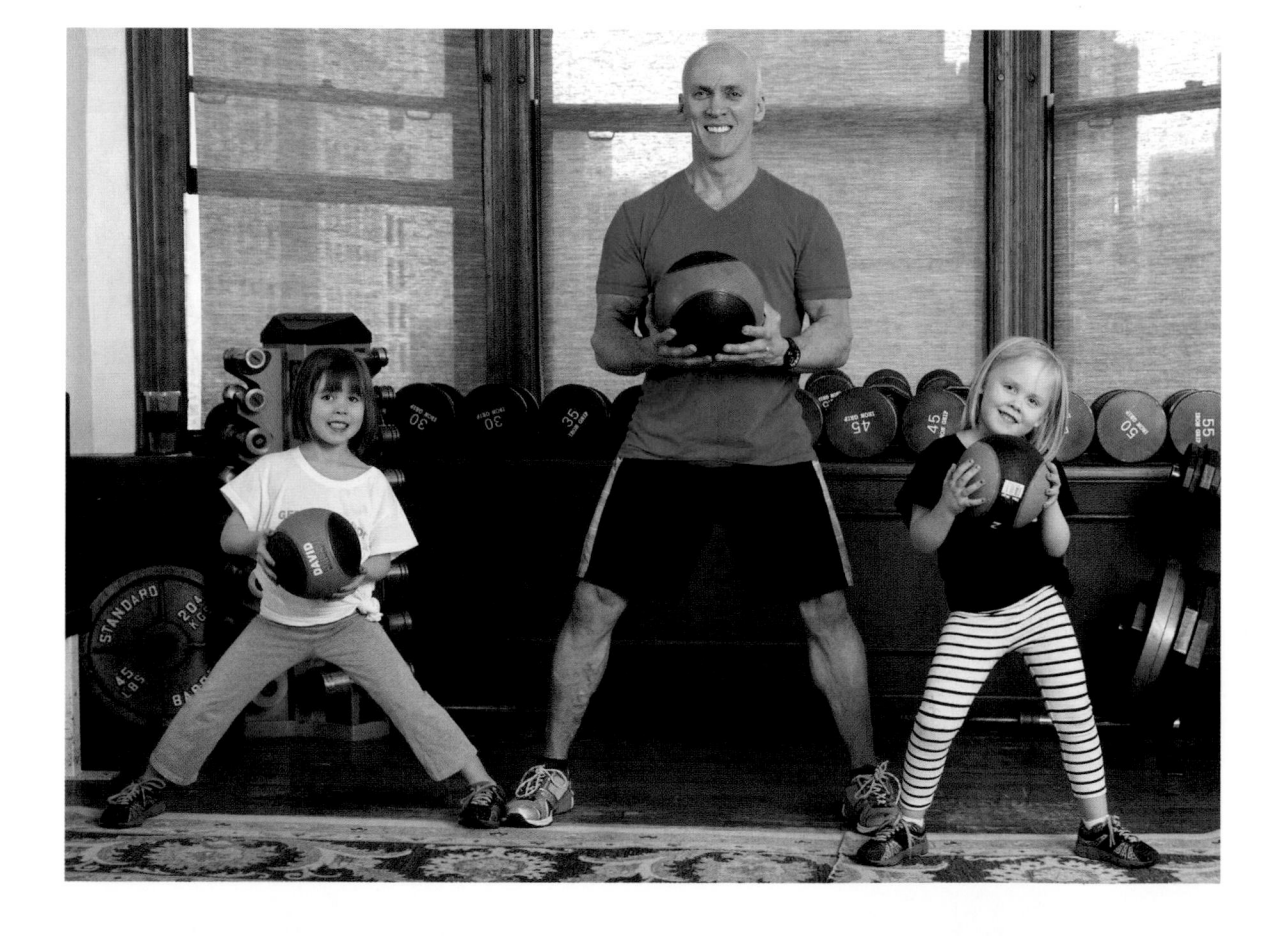

Lower Body	
Day 1	**1.** Sumo lunges to a side kick with squat jumps *p. 36*
	2. Single leg deadlifts *p.38*
	3. Plié toe squats *p. 38*
	4. Reverse crossover lunge to lateral lunge *p. 40*
	5. Switch lunges *p. 42*
Day 2	**1.** Platypus walks *p. 44*
	2. Reverse lunge to high kick *p. 47*
	3. Stability ball scissors *p. 48*
	4. Single-leg bridges on a medicine ball *p. 50*
	5. Jump squats *p. 50*
Day 3	**1.** Forward and reverse lunges *p. 52*
	2. Single-leg squats with a stability ball *p. 54*
	3. One-legged squats into seesaws *p. 55*
	4. Hamstring curls with a stability ball *p. 56*
	5. Lateral lunge to a hip abduction *p. 57*
Day 4	**1.** Sumo lunges to a side kick with squat jumps *p. 36*
	2. Platypus walks *p. 44*
	3. Reverse crossover lunge to lateral lunge *p. 40*
	4. Jump squats *p. 50*
	5. Single leg squats with stability ball *p. 54*
Day 5	**1.** Single leg deadlifts *p. 38*
	2. Plié toe squats *p. 38*
	3. Forward and reverse lunges *p. 52*
	4. One-legged squats into seesaws *p. 55*
	5. Switch lunges *p. 42*

Upper Body		
Day 1	**1.** Jumping jacks with shoulder presses *p. 58*	
	2. Burpees with a medicine ball *p. 60*	
	3. Mountain climbers with a medicine ball *p. 62*	
	4. Shadow boxing (with dumbbells or water bottles) *p. 64*	
	5. Stability ball pushups to knee tuck *p. 66*	
Day 2	**1.** Pushups with a hip extension *p. 72*	
	2. Stability ball handoffs *p. 74*	
	3. Jumping jacks with lateral and front raises *p. 76*	
	4. Plank with torso rotation to T-stand *p. 70*	
	5. Diamond pushups *p. 78*	
Day 3 (Express Plank Workout)	**1.** Plank with knee tuck to hip abduction *p. 98*	
	2. Plank with dumbbell row to triceps extension *p. 100*	
	3. Plank with front raise to side lateral *p. 102*	
	4. Side plank oblique crunches *p. 69*	
	5. Plank with shoulder taps *p. 104*	
Day 4	**1.** Jumping jacks with shoulder presses *p. 58*	
	2. Burpees with a medicine ball *p. 60*	
	3. Mountain climbers with a medicine ball *p. 62*	
	4. Stability ball diamond pushups to a knee tuck *p. 66*	
	5. Walking planks *p. 68*	
Day 5	**1.** Shadow boxing (with dumbbells or water bottles) *p. 64*	
	2. Jumping jacks with lateral and front raises *p. 76*	
	3. Walking planks *p. 68*	
	4. Stability ball handoffs *p. 74*	
	5. Plank with torso rotation to T-Stand *p. 70*	

Upper and Lower-Body Exercises	
Day 1	**1.** Around the world with a medicine ball *p. 80*
	2. Platypus walks with medicine ball overhead *p. 82*
	3. Medicine ball wood chop to a lateral lunge *p. 89*
	4. Squat with dumbbell overhead *p. 84*
	5. Switch lunges with a medicine ball overhead *p. 86*
Day 2	**1.** Forward and reverse lunge with a medicine ball overhead *p. 90*
	2. Burpees with Spiderman pushups *p. 92*
	3. Stability ball pike with a knee tuck *p. 94*
	4. Plié toe squats with lateral raises *p. 96*
	5. Wheelbarrow planks *p. 88*
Day 3 (Express Plank Workout)	**1.** Plank with knee tuck to hip abduction *p. 98*
	2. Plank with dumbbell row to triceps extension *p. 100*
	3. Plank with front raise to side lateral *p. 102*
	4. Side plank oblique crunches *p. 104*
	5. Plank with shoulder taps *p. 104*
Day 4	**1.** Shadow boxing (with deep wide stance squats) *p. 64*
	2. Spiderman crawls *p. 97*
	3. Platypus walks with a medicine ball overhead *p. 82*
	4. Sumo lunge with a medicine ball overhead *p. 36*
	5. Switch lunges (with a medicine ball overhead) *p. 86*
Day 5	**1.** Around the world with a medicine ball *p. 80*
	2. Stability ball pike with a knee tuck *p. 94*
	3. Wheelbarrow planks *p. 88*
	4. Burpees with a medicine ball *p. 60*
	5. Jump squats with a medicine ball overhead *p. 50*

Five-Day Meal Tracker

This tracker provides you with recommended meals for the five-day plan. You can substitute other five-day approved recipes from chapter 4 to suit your dietary needs or restrictions and your personal tastes. Be sure you eat two snacks and three meals every day, drink plenty of water, and enjoy.

	Day 1	Day 2	Day 3	Day 4	Day 5
Breakfast*	Spinach & Egg Kirsch Muffins (page 148)	Bacon, Egg and Cheese Wrap (page 151)	Roasted Red Pepper Kirsch Egg Muffins (page 152)	Bacon, Egg and Cheese Wrap (page 151)	Crunchy Lettuce Tofu Tacos (page 157)
Snack	Approved Snack	Approved Snack	Approved Snack	Approved Snack	Approved Snack
Lunch	Tuna Spinach Bowl (page 173)	Sauteed Collard Greens with Lentils (page 182)	Grilled Vegetable Wrap with Hummus (page 159)	Crunchy Romaine Avocado Salad (page 184)	Chicken Noodle Soup (page 169)
Snack	Approved Snack	Approved Snack	Approved Snack	Approved Snack	Approved Snack
Dinner	Turkey Kale Soup (page 169)	Grilled Turkey Burgers with Cauliflower Mash (page 170)	Steamed Fish in Parchment (page 181)	Crispy Salmon Nuggets (page 177)	Chicken Cashew Stir-Fry (page 174)

*If you're short on time, you have a protein smoothie on the go for breakfast. See recipes on pages 144 and 146.

Approved snack list:

- Handful of nuts such as almonds, walnuts, or pistachios
- Bell pepper
- Cucumbers
- Celery
- Hard-boiled egg

Five-Day Cheat Sheet

These lists will give you the dos and don'ts of the five-day plan at a glance.

A-Okay

- Lean proteins such as turkey and chicken breast, nuts, fish, and tofu; seitan, beans, lentils, and quinoa if you're vegetarian
- Vegetables such as kale, spinach, broccoli, Brussels sprouts, chard, cauliflower, celery, cabbage, asparagus, and cucumbers
- Eggs
- Herbs and spices
- Avocado
- Alliums such as garlic, onions, and shallots
- Nuts such as walnuts, almonds, and pistachios

No Way

- Alcohol
- Processed and refined foods such as pasta, bread, crackers, cookies, etc.
- Carbohydrates, including starchy vegetables such as potatoes and corn
- Sugar
- Artificial sweeteners
- Fruits and berries
- Dairy
- Grains

FIVE RULES TO LIVE BY

By now you know how to eat and exercise for the five-day plan as well as for life. I will now share my five rules to living a happy, balanced, "well" life. Don't short-change yourself. My Ultimate Family Wellness Plan is not just a quick-fix weight loss diet plan; it is a wellness and lifestyle family guide. The following rules will help to galvanize your mind and spirit from the inside out, as the exercise and nutrition components of the plan strengthen you from the outside in.

In the rest of this chapter, you'll learn how to live in the moment, be accountable, avoid—or at least deal with—stressful situations, believe in yourself, and incorporate healthy living, eating, and exercise into your daily routine. I cannot stress enough the importance of incorporating movement and exercise and making healthy food choices. Make these as much a daily ritual as washing your face and brushing your teeth. When looked at that way, healthy living—through eating and exercise—is hard to live without.

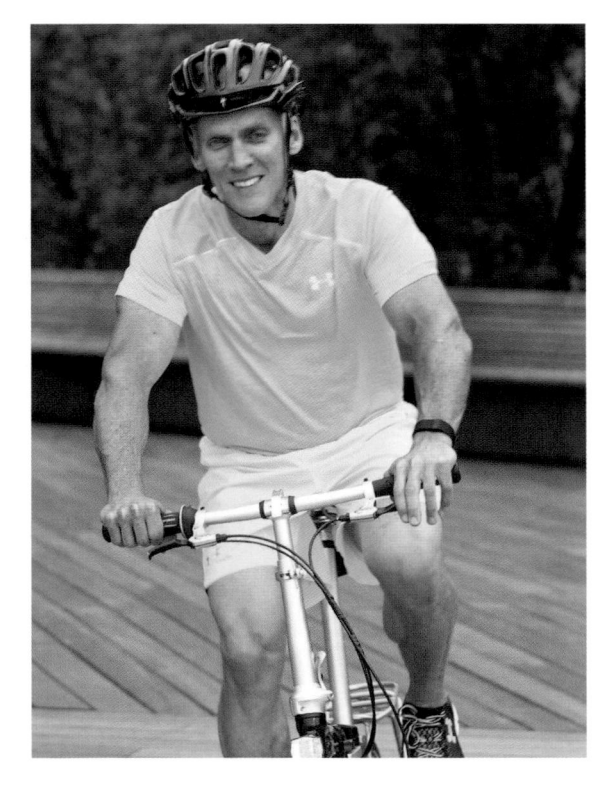

RULE 1: Live in the moment.

We all know people stuck in the past or planning for the future. I'll often sit with friends and clients, stalled in their wellness programs, mired in the past. To live a healthy, balanced, productive life, you need to live in the present and say to yourself, "Today is the first day of the rest of my life." The saying isn't "Tomorrow is the first day . . . ."

I like to look at the past as a series of teaching moments that guide us to where we are and should be in our lives. Carrying the past around like a ball and chain serves no one, least of all, you. While living in the future, "I'm going to start eating better and exercising tomorrow," opens up that procrastination box. There are so many tomorrows and only one today. Seize the moment now—be all that you can be this very moment. As I've often heard and said, there is no better time than now. No one knows what tomorrow will bring, so, as the proverb says, "Don't put off until tomorrow what you can do today."

RULE 2: Be accountable.

It seems like a simple concept yet it often eludes us. How many times do we say to ourselves, "If only he didn't stress me out so much, I wouldn't have eaten the pint of ice cream," or, "I would've worked out, but the kids had a rough night and kept me up." Look, I've been there. As a single father of five-year-old girls, I have had my share of sleepless, restless nights, stressful, shortened workdays, and too little time for a proper workout. As an entrepreneur and small business owner, I often get pulled in so many directions that finding "me time" seems an impossible task. I don't always have the answer, nor do I always do the right thing, but I refuse to be a passive victim. I own and try to learn from my mistakes.

As parents, we raise our children to be accountable, tell the truth, know right from wrong, and when necessary, have the courage and strength to apologize. As a parent, I like to lead by example and hold myself up to an even stricter standard. There have definitely been times when I've said to Emilia and Francesca, "Daddy was wrong for saying or doing _____, and he's sorry." You'll find that accountability is ultimately empowering as it will give you a higher sense of self, which will help enable you to stay the course on your health and wellness program.

RULE 3: Believe in yourself.

"Believe in yourself and all that you are. Know that there is something inside you that is greater than any obstacle."

—Christian D. Larson

I am raising Emilia and Francesca with these invaluable tenets. I take great pride and pleasure in listening to my daughters speak Mandarin to each other, ski, play tennis, chess, and piano, and handle difficult situations with grace, poise, and confidence. They are far from perfect, but they do their best, and in so doing, embrace the power of possibility. We can accomplish anything we set our minds and hearts to.

I try to instill that same level of confidence in my clients in our initial consultations and throughout our work together. Successfully completing this program will instill a renewed self-confidence and belief in your abilities.

"We are who we believe we are."

—C. S. Lewis

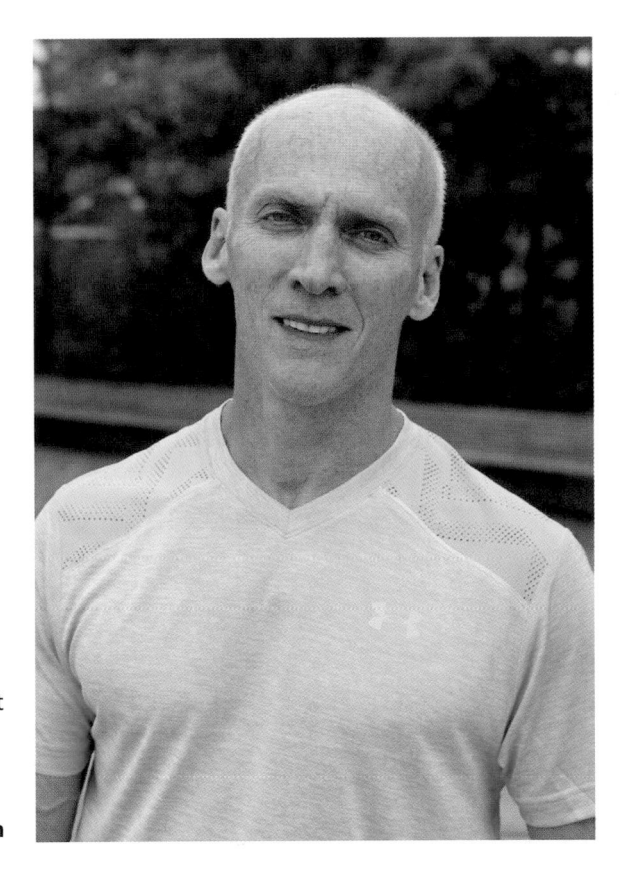

RULE 4: Don't let stress sabotage wellness goals.

Stress has been the undoing of many diets and exercise plans. In the name of transparency, I must say, that being a single father of twin girls, though immensely rewarding, can be incredibly stressful at times. I'd like to share with you some of my stress-busting tips:

Five deep breaths. The power of five deep breaths will help diffuse even the most stressful moments. Trust me, I have those days when the stars are not aligned anywhere in my life. It took me awhile to learn how to deal with really stressful situations and realizing the power of breathing—allowing that moment to collect yourself—helps immeasurably. I found a quote from a Chinese adage that I really love and want to share with you: "If you know the art of breathing you have the strength, wisdom, and courage of ten tigers."

Visualization. Find that happy place. When something is stressful, try to remove yourself mentally and physically. Whether it's the tender moment you had with your partner, child, or friend, a special place you visited and loved, or something extraordinary you did, call upon those moments when you need a mental or spiritual lift.

Exercise. There have been times, too numerous to recall, when a simple set of pushups helped me reconnect to my inner self, calm, and ground me. I learned this from my father, as he would often descend to his "inner sanctum," his makeshift gym in my childhood home, at the end of a long workday or after a stressful moment in the house. Well, the apple didn't fall too far from the tree.

Exercise has been the prescription for most that ails me. It has de-stressed me, healed me, and empowered me. Remember, pushups aren't for everyone. Don't underestimate the power of

walking and moving your body. I watch the effect it has on Emilia and Francesca when, after a long day at school, they head (rather sprint) to gymnastics or soccer. We can all learn from our children; running around and "letting off steam" is good and healthy.

RULE 5: Connect mind and body.

The final rule to live by applies to the exercise we do and the foods we eat. Being mindful of how and what you eat and whether and what you do for exercise will help guide and enlighten you on the path to total wellness. What goes on inside your head is just as important as the food you eat and the exercises you complete. To maintain the results you get with this or any program, you must make a deep internal change that will flip your motivation switch, helping you stay on your wellness program for the rest of your life. That change will involve, among other things, sound thinking.

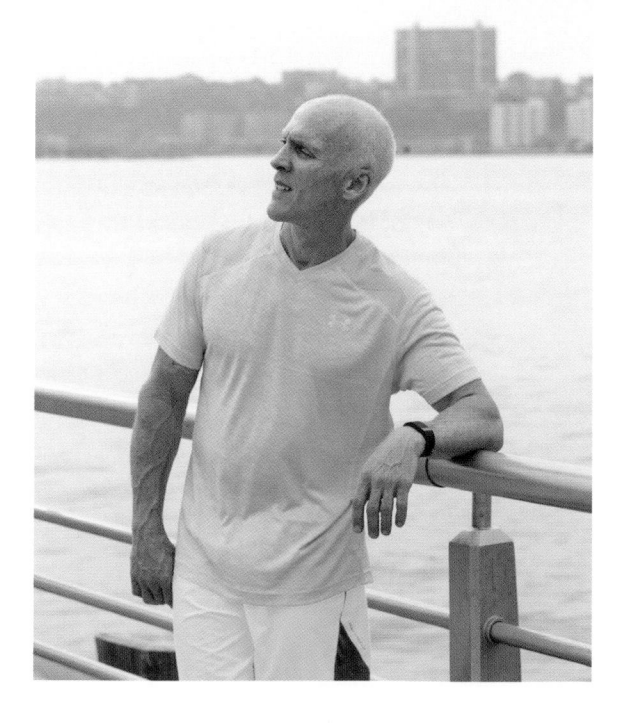

For example, do your emotions affect your eating? Do you eat when you are angry, sad, frustrated, or stressed? Do you get so stressed out at work that you have no energy to exercise afterwards? Are you sometimes so depressed that you can't motivate yourself to get off the couch? If you don't address the reason you eat the way you do or the way you live your life, you won't be able to maintain your results well past this intense five-day program.

The 5-5-5 Program is physically and mentally challenging. To be successful, you will need inner strength and the belief that you can do anything you set your mind to. Simply put, what you believe influences what you will accomplish. Here are some helpful tips:

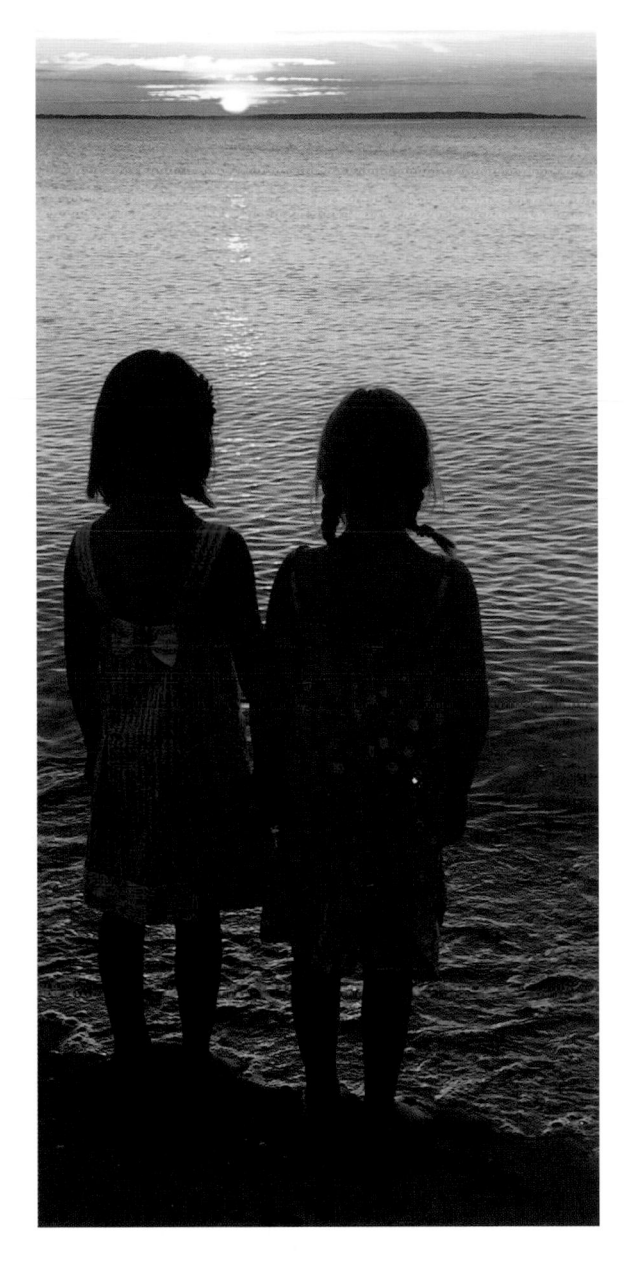

- Stay in touch with you. Keep a journal of your thoughts, feelings, and physical accomplishments.

- Find your motivation. Define the reason(s) you are doing this program. This will help keep you on track.

- Make exercise a daily ritual. Like washing your face and brushing your teeth, exercise must become part of your daily to-do list.

- Eat to live; don't live to eat. Fuel to move and function and not to mindlessly indulge. Start to look at food as fuel for your body and stick to premium, unprocessed foods. Listen to your belly, as I've taught Emilia and Francesca to do. Ask yourself, "Am I really hungry?"

- Be comfortable with failure. Don't let the fear of failing prevent you from attaining your goals.

- Stay positive. Accept that you can and will be the best you can be. Embrace your demons and learn to turn lemons into lemonade.

- Redesign your life for success. Your home, kitchen, pantry, family, and supportive friends should all be active parts of achieving our goals.

Getting a handle on your inner world can help create more energy for your wellness program.

MAINTENANCE

You have just completed the five-day portion of the Ultimate Family Wellness Program and accomplished what you previously thought was unattainable. Not only have you dropped at least five pounds and reshaped your body in just five days, you have started to transform your life, your family, and your home into the Ultimate Wellness Family. In five days, you were able to break down obstacles that may have prevented you from successfully realizing your goals in the past—lack of time for exercise, family stress and demands, no time to cook wholesome delicious meals. But, as is the case with all of my programs, the real takeaway is the knowledge and confidence you have gained in yourself and your ability to maintain and improve upon your results. Here are a few key points:

- You now have a greater understanding of how and when to prepare wholesome meals for your family, all while staying optimally fueled for your new-and-improved wellness lifestyle.

- You understand the importance of making yourself a priority and looking at exercise and movement for you and your family as a daily ritual (like on cold days when I force the issue and Emilia, Francesca, and I walk to school and check out "our" 25th Street winter garden).

- You have a better understanding of your body and know how to improve upon your pet peeves.

The last part is a wellness quotient test. Ask yourself the following questions:

1 How do you perceive yourself now?

2 How do you think other people perceive you?

3 Do you have the courage and confidence to motivate, inspire, and lead your family (and others) to a healthier, more active lifestyle?

4 What were your goals for the program?

5 What are they now? At some point during the past five days, you probably experienced the realization that your true goals had more to do with pushing yourself (and your family) to its fullest potential and less to do with looking like a super model or hero.

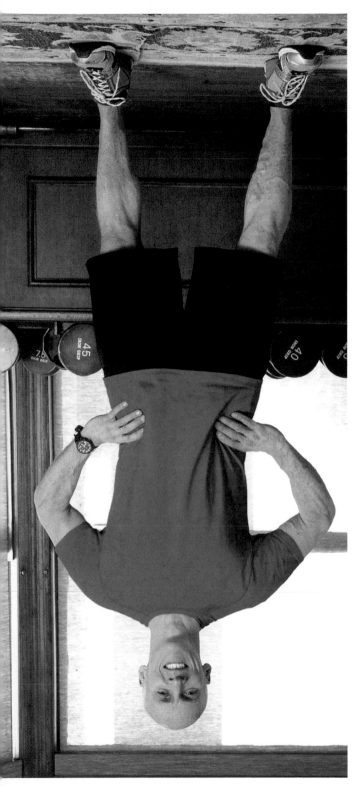

6 How has your attitude toward food and healthy family meals changed? You won't always eat perfectly, but you will make smarter choices, and when you do indulge in that occasional treat (e.g., gelato or a biscotti), you and your family will savor the moment.

7 How has your attitude toward life changed? Your and your family's life is more healthful, you have learned to prioritize, and you have learned that a little bit of movement, every day, is something for which to strive.

As for maintaining and building on the results of the previous five days, it is quite simple: Keep doing what you're doing. I don't mean exercising every day or always abstaining from your favorite treats and indulgences. Rather, now that you have a more enlightened understanding of how seamless it is to embrace small snippets of exercise throughout your day and now that you have the tools and confidence to prepare and create your own unique fast, delicious, and nutritious recipes, you will be able to confidently stay the wellness course. Your five-day jump-start program has not only yielded amazing physical results, but in the process, has transformed you and your family for life.

ACKNOWLEDGMENTS

This book has been a labor of love! I have several people I want to thank for their contributions and tireless support. First and foremost, I would like to thank the co-stars and inspiration behind this book—my daughters, Emilia and Francesca. You fill my heart and my life with endless love, pride, and pleasure that calms delights and empowers me! I am so proud of both of you and can't imagine my life without you! Whether helping me to create new and exciting recipes; three days of tireless energy photo shoots; inspiring me to get up and move on those lazy mornings; or patiently understanding that "daddy needed to finish a chapter." Your love, support, and patience on those late nights, early mornings, and weekends, helped make this book more than just a dream—you helped it come to life! How many animals are we going to have on our farm? To my friends Kathryn, owner of Agency 4 Surrogacy, and Michele for helping me realize the dream of fatherhood by being our gestational carrier. I am eternally grateful!

I would like to thank my dear friend Marcus for his belief in me and for always telling me like it is, even when I didn't necessarily want to hear it. He also introduced me to my publisher, Winnie, who from our first meeting in my office, I immediately connected with. After accepting my proposal for my 5-5-5 Program, she didn't waiver when I told her I wanted to write more than just a fitness book. Thank you for letting me share my personal journey and evolution from being a celebrity trainer to a family fitness/wellness parent of twin girls—and how that impacted how I look at fitness and wellness. Winnie, John, Katie, Regina, Mary, and the entire team at Fair Winds Press—it has been a pleasure and an honor being one of your authors. To Luciana for her beautiful photography! Your keen eye caught the essence of the message of the book—good health and wellness is fun and accessible at any age!

Katherine, thank you for helping me organize, edit, and make sense of the many thoughts, words, and ideas that are in this book. It was really a pleasure working with you!

When I decided to write this book and knew there would be a food component, I reached out to my very dear friend Jennifer, who as in the past, tasted, tested, critiqued, and—when need be—tweaked each and every recipe in the book. Thank you and Alan for your love and for always being there! I am so grateful to have you in my life.

To my friend Heidi and her team at Krupp Kommunications for their tireless efforts, and Susan and the PR team at Trachtenberg for years of great work and for helping create buzz, press, and media for this book and me.

This past year has been a particularly difficult one for my family and me. I am so grateful to be surrounded by a loving, caring, and strong family. Mom and Dad—I am especially proud of you for the courage, strength, and dignity you have showed throughout. What an incredible teaching moment for all who love you—especially for Emilia and Francesca—we love you so very much! To my sister and most importantly, my best friend, Bonnie—words minimize.

To my staff and trainers and members of the Madison Square Club—thank you for helping keep my dream alive. I had a dream twenty-five years ago, and I am proud to say that with your help and loyalty we have helped transform thousands of lives.

I want to thank Jennifer for her kind and thoughtful foreword and Liv, Kate, Danny, Jeff, and Joy for not only their beautiful words, but also for their friendship and support. It really means the world to me.

Last but not least, I want to thank you for indulging me and letting me share Emilia, Francesca, and my story. You have showed us love, kindness, and support for which we will be eternally grateful!

In Good Health

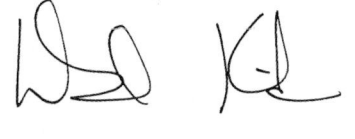

ABOUT THE AUTHOR

With over two decades of experience uncovering and harnessing the powerful connection between mind, body, and spirit, David Kirsch has become a leading authority on achieving optimal health and well-being at any age or fitness level. Throughout his years as a sought-after trainer, David has transformed the bodies—and lives—of countless devotees through his signature combination of mind-body conditioning, multi-tasking workouts, and smart nutrition. From founding New York's award-winning Madison Square Club to developing unprecedented supplements, classes, and techniques designed to maximize workouts, David has been a pioneer in the wellness field throughout his long career.

Trusted by some of the world's most visible celebrities and influencers, David is the man with whom many A-listers train when they need to get in shape fast. One of the unique aspects of training with David is his expertise in reading different body types and his ability to target different parts of the body. In addition to authoring five books, including the bestseller *The Ultimate New York Body Plan*, David has appeared on numerous television shows, including The *Today Show*, E! and *CNN World News*, *Dr. Oz*, *Live with Regis and Kelly*, and *The View*. Additionally, as a single father of five-year-old twin girls, he has expanded his wellness empire to include areas such as family and child fitness, nutrition, and wellness. His website, DavidKirschWellness.com, represents a passport to the complete David Kirsch lifestyle.

Get Kirsched!

http://davidkirschwellness.com

http://about.me/davidkirsch

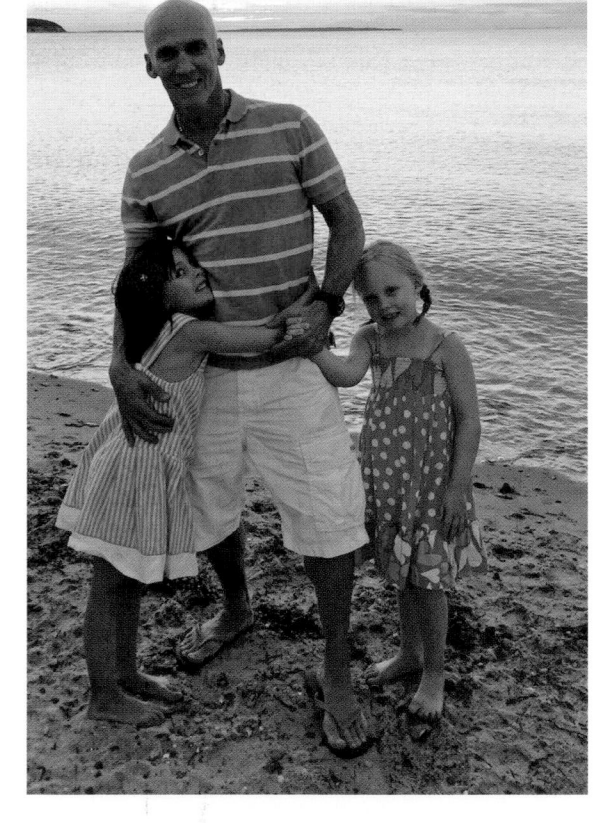

RESOURCES

CREATING THE ULTIMATE FAMILY WELLNESS HOME

Over the years, I have tried and tested many different brands of foods—from beverages to cooking sprays, condiments, and basic pantry staples. I have found that the key to maintaining a healthy, balanced home is to have your favorite products readily available in your pantry, and in certain cases, your personal vanity. From my favorite pasta to my favorite skin-firming cream, the following is a comprehensive, though not totally exhaustive, list:

Products for your ultimate family wellness–

Food

- **Andean Dream**—This is another healthy alternative to pasta and is made with the delicious superfood quinoa. www.andeandream.com

- **Banza**—My daughters and I love eating this pasta because it is a healthier alternative to traditional pasta. Banza is gluten-free and made with high-protein chickpeas. www.eatbanza.com

- **Fig Food Company**—Beans are an important staple in my family's daily diet and there is nothing better than having ready-to-eat organic beans. www.figfood.com

- **Tolerant**—This is a delicious pasta made from red or black beans. It is a great gluten-free substitute that doesn't sacrifice on taste. www.tolerantfoods.com

- **Pomi chopped tomatoes, puree, and paste**—When tomatoes are out of season, I rely on Pomi to more than satisfactorily fill in. www.pomi.us.com

- **Sauces 'n Love**—These highest quality sauces perfectly complement my healthy pasta dinners.

I also love that the sauces are gluten-free and all-natural. www.saucesnlove.com

- **Success**—I like to keep a couple of boxes of this "instant" brown rice around, as it's great if you are running short on time and want a healthy, gluten-free snack. www.successrice.com

- **Bob's Red Mill**—Bob's Red Mill sells delicious grains that I use often, including their gluten-free oats and almond flour. I also like the rolled oats, which I use in my turkey burgers. www.bobsredmill.com

- **Canyon Bakehouse**—I prefer serving Emilia and Francesca gluten–free bread, and I choose this as my go-to brand —it's delicious as well as whole grain. www.canyonglutenfree.com

- **Damascus Bakeries**—They know health and carbs do not necessarily go together, so they offer a healthy solution: flat bread. I use their great tasting flax roll-ups for my breakfast wraps. www.damascusbakery.com

- **Sir Kensington's**—This is my favorite Dijon mustard. From adding zip to my morning eggs, to adding extra flavor to my turkey burgers, I use it in everything—just ask my girls! www.sirkensingtons.com

- **Traina**—I love the sun-dried fruit Traina creates; it is truly a delicious snack. My daughters and I also love it in our sauces, sautés, and salads. www.trainafoods.com

- **True Made Foods**—I love this ketchup because it is created with all organic vegetables such as squash, spinach, and carrots, yet still tastes delicious. www.truemadefoods.com

- **La Tourengelle**—I love these oils because they are created by an authentic and traditional family producer in both France and California. I particularly like the walnut oil—with its high level of omega 3 and 6's and its delicious flavor. I love using it when making my special vegetable stir-fry. www.latourangelle.com

- **Spectrum**—I love the convenience of having healthy, organic spray oils for cooking. My favorites are olive oil, grapeseed, and safflower. www.spectrumorganics.com

- **The Olive Fruit**—This is my choice for olive oil, and I use it to add some flavor to my dishes. www.theolivefruit.com

- **Applegate Naturals**—This is my go-to source for turkey bacon and I like that they produce healthy meat that is raised humanely without antibiotics or hormones. www.applegate.com

- **Tonnino**—My family loves Tonnino Tuna because it mixes delicious yellow-fin and other wild-fin tuna with great flavors. www.tonnino.com

- **Pillar Rock**—Delicious packaged salmon that is convenient to use. It is readily available and is a pantry essential. www.oceanbeauty.com/retail-brands

- **Cholula Hot Sauce**—This is a delicious hot sauce that is not too spicy but also not too mild. It is a perfect balance of heat and flavor that I really enjoy. My eggs would seem naked without it! www.cholula.com

- **David's Kosher Salt**—A versatile kosher salt that is great for everyday cooking because of its coarse and flaky texture. www.davidskosher.com

- **Simply Organic**—My go-to for when I am not able to get fresh organic herbs. I love that they offer food made for a person who is passionate about health and wellness. www.simplyorganic.com

- **Truvia**—A zero-calorie, all-natural sweetener made from the stevia plant that I love to use in my tea and when preparing some healthy snacks with Emilia and Francesca. http://truvia.com

- **Xochitl**—This is a great salsa that I use for snacks because it is delicious and made with all-natural vegetables and ingredients. www.salsaxochitl.com

- **Freedom Foods**—I like Freedom Foods because they work with artisan food producers to authentically deliver all-natural and delicious products. www.freedom-foods.com

- **Navitas**—This is my go-to brand for chia seeds, hemp seeds, cacao nibs, maca and green coffee powder, which are all important parts of my diet. I use Navitas for my seeds because they are naturally produced with minimal processing and are high quality. www.navitasnaturals.com

- **The Splendid Spoon**—I love the Splendid Spoon because they offer a different perspective on soups; they are made with all-natural, organic ingredients that can be consumed on-the-go. I really enjoy the convenience of grabbing one and drinking it as a quick and healthy snack or lunch. www.thesplendidspoon.com/#newdrinkablecleanse

- **Fage**—My family's Greek yogurt of choice because it is high in protein and healthy. http://usa.fage.eu

- **Nutiva**—I love to use their organic buttery spread on my daughters' French toast, in place of butter. It is created from a delicious blend of red palm oil and virgin coconut oil. www.nutiva.com

Health and Beauty

Optimal health, beauty, and wellness is not only about the foods we eat, but also the products we use to nourish and protect our skin, face, and body. Here are some of my favorites:

- **Nerium Firm**—The ultimate firming and toning cream to target problem areas such as stomach, arms, and thighs. www.nerium.com

- **Colbert MD** –My daily regimen for nutritious and healthy skin. I love to use the serum and the illumino oil every day. www.colbertmd.com

- **Baum De Rose by Terry**—The most amazing nutria regenerating lip balm. My go-to for keeping my lips and nails healthy and hydrated. www.byterry.com

- **Kiss My Face**—I love this natural mineral sunscreen because it is made with nourishing oils, vitamins, and great antioxidants. I keep plenty on hand for Emilia, Francesca, and myself. www.kissmyface.com

- **EOS**—A great lip balm that nourishes and replenishes vital nutrients and vitamins to the lips. My daughters' favorite lip balm; they love the different flavors. www.evolutionofsmooth.com

- **Under Armour**—State-of-the-art athletic apparel that men, women, and even children can wear to enhance athletic performance. www.underarmour.com/en-us

- **Athos**—I love Athos athletic gear because it allows the wearer to track his or her own heart rate, breathing rate, and even what muscles are being targeted during exercise. www.liveathos.com

Hydration

Staying hydrated is ever so important, so when the girls and I are not drinking water, here are some of our favorite beverage treats.

- **Andros**—They have a delicious apple juice squeeze that is all-natural and does not contain any added sugar. www.andros.com.cn

- **Drink Blocks**—A fun and playful way for my kids to stay hydrated. These drinks are sugar-free, zero-calorie, naturally flavored waters that are also building blocks ready to be played with. www.drinkblocks.com

- **Harvest Bay**—They not only offer delicious coconut water, but also a great, easy-to-use coconut oil spray that is a kitchen necessity. www.harvest-bay.com

- **Harmless Harvest** – Delicious coconut water that is 100-percent raw. I love that the brand stays true to their high standard of quality beverages. Emilia loves that the coconut water has a pink hue. www.harmlessharvest.com

- **ITO EN**—ITO EN tea is a terrific bottled green tea and I like that the company upholds their products to the principles of being healthy, natural, and safe. www.itoen.com

- **Jax Coco**—I love the convenience of the small Jax Coco beverages. They are great snacks for my daughters, and I love blending them in shakes with my David Kirsch vitamin drinks. www.jaxcoco.com

- **Mamma Chia**—My daughters, Emelia and Francesca, absolutely love this drink, and I do too because it has 1,200mg of healthy omega-3s. www.mammachia.com

- **Peter Rabbit Organics**—Another great-tasting vegetable and fruit squeeze that does not contain any added sugar. www.peterrabbitorganics.com

Snacks

Snacking is not a bad thing—we all love to do it! The following are some of Emilia and Francesca's favorite go-to snacks:

- **Beanfield**—I love these healthy chips because they are delicious and plant-based, non-GMO snacks with beans as the primary ingredient. www.beanfieldssnacks.com

- **Bearitos**—Another great-tasting chip brand that is made with all-natural ingredients and contains no artificial flavors or preservatives. www.bearitos.com

- **Emmy's**—I love these delicious treats because they are vegan, gluten-free and made with high-quality raw ingredients. www.emmysorganics.com

- **Dang**—These all-natural coconut chips are made with delicious flavors and are another staple in my girls' snack bags. www.dangfoods.com

- **Gim Me Organic**—This is Emilia's go-to afternoon snack! I love these delicious seaweed snacks because they are packed with important vitamins and minerals. www.gimmehealth.com

- **I Heart Keenwah**—These snacks are an easy, healthy, and delicious treat and are created with the superfood, quinoa. www.iheartkeenwah.com

- **Mary's Gone Crackers**—I love these organic, gluten-free vegan crackers, pretzels, and cookies. www.marysgonecrackers.com

- **Nelly's**—A delicious pick-me-up snack that my daughters' love—and I love that it is only made with organic ingredients. www.nellysorganics.com

- **Next Organics**—These delicious and organic dark chocolate snacks are a perfect combination of healthy dark chocolate, nuts, and fruits. I am especially addicted to the dark chocolate espresso beans. www.nextchocolates.com

- **Pipcorn**—I find these small kernels to be a perfect gluten-free vegan snack for my daughters. They love it! www.pipsnacks.com

- **Seapoint Farms**—Perfect for both children and adults, I love that these are not only delicious but also made with non-GMO soybeans. www.seapointfarms.com

- **Snacks 101**—I love to give my girls this popcorn because it is whole grain, gluten-free and delicious. www.snacks101.com

- **You love Fruit**—These snacks are made from 100-percent real fruit and contain no artificial flavors or preservatives. It is a healthy and delicious staple in my daughters' snack bags. www.fruitspotz.com

- **T- Fal ActiFry**—Who doesn't love french fries? I love to use my air fryer to cook healthy french fries for my daughters—made with just one tablespoon (15 ml) of grapeseed oil. www.tfalactifry.com

- **All-Clad**—You can make really healthy meals with a slow cooker. I love using mine for a batch of turkey chili, for instance. www.all-clad.com

- **Vitamix Blenders**—My smoothies and soups would be lost without my Vitamix Professional Series 750. It has five pre-programmed settings, speed controls, and other features for high-performance blending. www.vitamix.com

- **Omega Juicer**—In addition to using my Vitamix blender, I use my Omega juicer to create my green beverages every morning. It is important to have fresh, healthy, and delicious juices as a nutritious aspect of your diet. www.omegajuicers.com

- **Thrive Market**—Thrive Market is an online shopping club where members can purchase a variety of food items, which can be especially helpful if there are limited products at food stores nearby. www.thrivemarket.com

Nutritional Supplements

During the course of the program (and ideally beyond) you are going to consume five meals a day, approximately every three hours. Your meals will consist of lean protein and fiber-rich vegetables and salad. If you are like me and most of my clients, finding the time to eat five meals a day can be as daunting as the idea of completing one of the five exercise circuits. I hate to admit it, but there are days when my best laid plan of five meals a day goes out the window by mid-morning snack! From getting Emilia and Francesca up, fed, and out to school, client sessions and other work related things, meals fall by the wayside. We all know how nutrition is such a key component to one's overall wellness. It is also a fact that breakfast is the most important meal of the day! Studies have shown that breakfast meals consisting of protein will keep you sated longer (and help take you hunger-free to your next meal).

Those of you that know me—either personally or from my previous books—or follow me on social media, know that I am a huge proponent of nutritional supplements. Over the years, I have tried and tasted myriad brands and their unique offerings. The supplements I use on a regular basis are whey protein powder, natural energy drinks, and multiple vitamins. I look for natural ingredients with no artificial flavors, colors, or sweeteners. If you're using a brand of supplements that meet those guidelines, then continue using them. If not, or if you want to try a premium natural supplements line, you may want to try David Kirsch Wellness One of a Kind Supplements®. I created One of a Kind Supplements—a natural line of health, wellness, and beauty supplements to address my and my clients' busy lifestyles and lack of time to always prepare the meals we consume. For this program, I have picked a set of five of my top-selling supplements and created the 5-5-5 Ultimate Wellness Kit™. I am not saying that taking my supplements is key to successfully completing the program, but it definitely won't hurt.

- **Protein Plus protein powder**—25 grams of whey protein isolate make this the perfect "breakfast on the run." I mix mine with almond milk, chia seeds, cacao nibs, and wheat germ, and love it as my breakfast, snack, or, on occasion, dinner.

- **Thermo, Energy, Calming**—the best–selling "Bubbles Trifecta" will help give you energy, help metabolize and burn fat and calories, curb your appetite, and keep you calm.

- **Vitamin Mineral Super Juice**—the box says it all: "drink your vitamins®!" Sugar-free natural-flavored vitamin sachets that turn ordinary water into a delicious, nutritious, and highly satisfying vitamin drink.

- **Afternoon Energy**—this capsule packs a potent proprietary blend of, among other things, tyrosine to help you improve your mood and your focus, and B12 for your immune system and energy.

- **Super Charged Greens**—for those times when a plate of spinach or broccoli is nary to be found; a comprehensive blend of fruits and greens extracts, probiotics and post–biotic, make this an invaluable product.

INDEX

action plans, 24, 31
adaptation, 16–17, 35, 107
alcohol, 117, 123
Almond-Lime Marinade
    Chicken Cashew Stir-Fry, 174
    recipe, 196
almonds
    Banana Chocolate Protein
      Smoothie, 144
    benefits of, 119, 132, 137
    as superfood, 137
    Tuna Spinach Bowl, 173
    Whole-Wheat Almond Pan-
      cakes, 154
anise, benefits of, 126
Apple Cider Vinaigrette
    Crunchy Romaine Avocado
      Salad, 184
    recipe, 194
apples
    Crunchy Romaine Avocado
      Salad, 184
    Grilled Turkey Burgers, 170
Around the World with a Medi-
    cine Ball, 80–81
artificial sweeteners, 118–119, 125
asparagus. See Farro with Pars-
    ley and Asparagus, 166
avocados
    Avocado Berry Smoothie, 145
    benefits of, 123, 130–131, 139
    Crunchy Lettuce Tofu
      Tacos, 157
    Crunchy Romaine Avocado
      Salad, 184
    Roasted Turkey Avocado
      Salad, 162
    as superfood, 139
    Tuna Spinach Bowl, 173

Bacon, Egg, and Cheese
    Wrap, 151
bananas
    Banana Chocolate Protein
      Smoothie, 144
    Oatmeal Banana Brulee, 153
basil, benefits of, 126
beans
    benefits of, 119, 124, 138
    My Brown Rice and Beans, 158
    Sauteed Collard Greens with
      Lentils, 182
    as superfood, 138
blackberries
    Berry Protein Blast, 145
    Best Berry Yogurt Parfait,
      The, 153
    as superfood, 136
blueberries
    Best Berry Yogurt Parfait,
      The, 153

    as superfood, 136
    Vegan Berry Smoothie, 146
body types, 30
Bok Choy with Maitake Mush-
    rooms, 188
Brazil nuts, 132
breads, 123–124
breakfast
    Bacon, Egg, and Cheese
      Wrap, 151
    Best Berry Yogurt Parfait,
      The, 153
    Crunchy Lettuce Tofu
      Tacos, 157
    introduction to, 148
    Oatmeal Banana Brulee, 153
    Roasted Red Pepper Kirsch
      Egg Muffins, 152
    Spinach Egg Kirsch
      Muffins, 148
    Whole-Wheat Almond Pan-
      cakes, 154
broccoli
    benefits of, 120, 137
    Crunchy Stir-Fry, 192
    as superfood, 137
Brussels sprouts
    benefits of, 120
    Kale Salad, 185
    Roasted Carrots and Squash
      with Fresh Thyme, 187
buckwheat, benefits of, 126
Burpees with a Medicine Ball,
    60–61
Burpees with Spiderman Push-
    ups, 92–93

cabbage. See Crunchy Stir-Fry, 192
cardio
    Five-Minute Cardio
      Circuits, 106
    Gauntlet machines, 107
    high-intensity interval train-
      ing (HIIT), 26
    jump rope, 106
    maximizing benefits of, 107
    rowing machine, 106
    rowing machines, 107
    treadmill, 106, 107
    Versa climbers, 107
carrots
    Crunchy Quinoa Salad, 161
    Grilled Turkey Burgers, 170
    Roasted Carrots and Squash
      with Fresh Thyme, 187
    Thai Ginger Sirloin Salad, 178
cashews
    benefits of, 119, 132
    Chicken Cashew Stir-Fry, 174
    as superfood, 137

cauliflower
    benefits of, 120, 138
    Cauliflower Mash, 185
    Crunchy Stir-Fry, 192
    Roasted Carrots and Squash
      with Fresh Thyme, 187
    as superfood, 138
cayenne pepper, benefits of, 126
cheese
    Bacon, Egg, and Cheese
      Wrap, 151
    Kale Salad, 185
    Roasted Red Pepper Kirsch
      Egg Muffins, 152
chia seeds
    benefits of, 119, 128
    Berry Protein Blast, 145
    Best Berry Yogurt Parfait,
      The, 153
chicken
    benefits of, 119
    Chicken Cashew Stir-Fry, 174
    Chicken Noodle Soup, 169
    Chicken Stock, 195
Chicken Stock
    Cauliflower Mash, 185
    Chicken Noodle Soup, 169
    recipe, 195
    Turkey Kale Soup, 169
chickpeas. See My Ultimate
    Low-Fat Hummus, 198
children
    accountability and, 209
    exercise and, 30, 115, 210
    herbs and spices and, 129
    sugar consumption, 119
    superfoods for, 139
cinnamon, benefits of, 126–127
circuits, 35, 106
Cleansing Green Juice, 146
core
    Diamond Pushups, 78–79
    engaging, 32, 33
    Forward and Reverse Lunge
      with a Medicine Ball Over-
      head, 90–91
    Jumping Jacks with Lateral
      and Front Raises, 76–77
    Jumping Jacks with Shoulder
      Presses, 58–59
    Medicine Ball Wood Chop to
      a Lateral Lunge, 89
    Mountain Climbers with a
      Medicine Ball, 62–63
    Platypus Walks with a Medi-
      cine Ball, 82–83
    Plié Toe Squats, 38
    Squat with One Dumbbell
      Overhead, 84–85

    Stability Ball Pike with a
      Knee Tuck, 94–95
    Stability Ball Pushups to
      Knee Tuck, 66–67
    Switch Lunges with a Medi-
      cine Ball Overhead, 86–87
    Walking Planks, 68
corn, benefits of, 134
Crispy Salmon Nuggets, 177
Crunchy Lettuce Tofu Tacos, 157
Crunchy Quinoa Salad, 161
Crunchy Romaine Avocado
    Salad, 184
Crunchy Stir-Fry, 192
cucumber
    Cleansing Green Juice, 146
    Grilled Vegetable Wrap, 159

dairy, 125
Diamond Pushups, 78–79
dill, benefits of, 127
dinner
    Chicken Cashew Stir-Fry, 174
    Crispy Salmon Nuggets, 177
    Grilled Turkey Burgers, 170
    introduction to, 170
    Sauteed Collard Greens with
      Lentils, 182
    Steamed Fish in Parchment,
      181
    Thai Ginger Sirloin Salad, 178
    Tuna Spinach Bowl, 173
distractions, 31, 107
dumbbells
    Jumping Jacks with Lateral
      and Front Raises, 76–77
    Jumping Jacks with Shoulder
      Presses, 58–59
    Plank with Dumbbell Row
      to Triceps Extension,
      100–101
    Plank with Front Raise to
      Side Lateral, 102–103
    Plié Toe Squats with Lateral
      Raises, 96
    Shadow Boxing, 64–65
    Squat with One Dumbbell
      Overhead, 84–85

eggs
    Bacon, Egg, and Cheese
      Wrap, 151
    benefits of, 119, 125, 131–
      132, 135, 136
    Farro with Parsley and Aspar-
      agus, 166
    Roasted Red Pepper Kirsch
      Egg Muffins, 152
    Spinach Egg Kirsch
      Muffins, 148
    as snack, 132

as superfood, 135–136
Whole-Wheat Almond Pancakes, 154
Zucchini Scallion Pancakes, 191
essentials
Almond Lime Marinade, 196
Apple Cider Vinaigrette, 194
Chicken Stock, 195
Ginger Soy Dressing, 194
introduction to, 194
My Ultimate Low-Fat Hummus, 198
Roasted Rosemary Sage Turkey Breast, 198
Strawberry Vinaigrette, 195
Tomato-Watermelon Salsa, 196
Express Full-Body Plank Workout
introduction to, 98
Plank with Dumbbell Row to Triceps Extension, 100–101
Plank with Front Raise to Side Lateral, 102–103
Plank with Knee Tuck to Hip Abduction, 98–99
Plank with Shoulder Taps, 104–105
Side Plank Oblique Crunches, 104

failure
action plans and, 31
diet and, 32
distractions and, 31
sleep and, 32
farro
benefits of, 126
Farro with Parsley and Asparagus, 166
fats, 120, 125
fiber, 120, 125
Five-Day Cheat Sheet, 207
Five-Day Exercise Tracker, 202–205
Five-Day Meal Tracker, 206
Five-Minute Cardio Circuits, 106
Five Rules for Optimal Nutrition
alcohol, 117
artificial sweeteners, 118–119
fiber, 120
introduction to, 116
leafy vegetables, 120
processed foods, 117–118
proteins, 119–120
refined foods, 117–118
sugars, 118–119
flaxseeds, 119, 128
flounder. See Steamed Fish in Parchment, 181
form, 32–33
Forward and Reverse Lunges, 52–53
Forward and Reverse Lunge with a Medicine Ball Overhead, 90–91

garlic, benefits of, 127
Gauntlet machines, 107

ginger, benefits of, 127
Ginger-Soy Dressing
Crunchy Stir-Fry, 192
recipe, 194
Thai Ginger Sirloin Salad, 178
Grilled Turkey Burgers, 170
Grilled Vegetable Wrap, 159

Hamstring Curls with a Stability Ball, 56
hazelnuts
benefits of, 119, 132
Kale Salad, 185
as superfood, 137
hemp seeds
benefits of, 119, 128
Vegan Berry Smoothie, 146
high-intensity interval training (HIIT), 26

jicama. See Crunchy Quinoa Salad, 161
juices. See smoothies and juices.
Jumping Jacks with Lateral and Front Raises, 76–77
Jumping Jacks with Shoulder Presses, 58–59
jump ropes, 106
Jump Squats, 50–51

kale
Cleansing Green Juice, 146
Kale Salad, 185
Turkey Kale Soup, 169
kiwi
benefits of, 139
as superfood, 139

Lateral Lunge to a Hip Abduction, 57
lettuce
benefits of, 134
Crunchy Lettuce Tofu Tacos, 157
Crunchy Romaine Avocado Salad, 184
lower body exercises
Five-Day Exercise Tracker, 203
Forward and Reverse Lunges, 52–53
Hamstring Curls with a Stability Ball, 56
introduction to, 36
Jump Squats, 50–51
Lateral Lunge to a Hip Abduction, 57
One-Legged Squats into Seesaws, 55
Platypus Walks, 44–45
Plié Toe Squats, 38–39
Reverse Crossover Lunge to Lateral Lunge, 40–41
Reverse Lunge to High Kick, 46–47
Single-Leg Bridges on a Medicine Ball, 50
Single Leg Deadlifts, 38
Single-Leg Squat with a Stability Ball, 54
Stability Ball Scissors, 48–49

Sumo Lunge to a Side Kick with a Squat Jump, 36–37
Switch Lunges, 42–43
lunch
Chicken Noodle Soup, 169
Crunchy Quinoa Salad, 161
Farro with Parsley and Asparagus, 166
Grilled Vegetable Wrap, 159
introduction to, 158
My Brown Rice and Beans, 158
Quinoa Spaghetti, 165
Roasted Turkey Avocado Salad, 162
Turkey Kale Soup, 169
lunges
form, 33
Forward and Reverse Lunges, 52–53
Forward and Reverse Lunge with a Medicine Ball Overhead, 90–91
Lateral Lunge to a Hip Abduction, 57
Reverse Crossover Lunge to Lateral Lunge, 40–41
Reverse Lunge to High Kick, 46–47
Sumo Lunge to a Side Kick with a Squat Jump, 36–37
Switch Lunges, 42–43
Switch Lunges with a Medicine Ball Overhead, 86–87

Madison Square Club, 9, 17, 23
maintenance, 213
mangos. See Avocado Berry Smoothie, 145
medicine balls
Around the World with a Medicine Ball, 80–81
Burpees with a Medicine Ball, 60–61
Forward and Reverse Lunge with a Medicine Ball Overhead, 90–91
Medicine Ball Wood Chop to a Lateral Lunge, 89
Mountain Climbers with a Medicine Ball, 62–63
Platypus Walks with a Medicine Ball, 82–83
Single-Leg Bridges on a Medicine Ball, 50
Switch Lunges with a Medicine Ball Overhead, 86–87
monounsaturated fats, 120
Mountain Climbers with a Medicine Ball, 62–63
mushrooms
Bok Choy with Maitake Mushrooms, 188
Cauliflower Mash, 185
Chicken Noodle Soup, 169
My Brown Rice and Beans, 158
My Ultimate Low-Fat Hummus, 198

oats
benefits of, 139

Grilled Turkey Burgers, 170
Oatmeal Banana Brulee, 153
as superfood, 139
One-Legged Squats into Seesaws, 55
oranges. See Crunchy Quinoa Salad, 161
oregano, benefits of, 127–128

parsley, benefits of, 128
peanut butter. See Berry Protein Blast, 145
phytochemicals, 124
pine nuts
benefits of, 119, 132
Roasted Turkey Avocado Salad, 162
as superfood, 137
pistachio nuts, 132, 137
planks
Plank with Dumbbell Row to Triceps Extension, 100–101
Plank with Front Raise to Side Lateral, 102–103
Plank with Knee Tuck to Hip Abduction, 98–99
Plank with Shoulder Taps, 104–105
Plank with Torso Rotation to T-Stand, 70–71
Side Plank Oblique Crunches, 69, 104
Walking Planks, 68
Wheelbarrow Planks, 88
Platypus Walks, 44–45
Platypus Walks with a Medicine Ball, 82–83
Plié Toe Squats, 38–39
Plié Toe Squats with Lateral Raises, 96
pomegranate seeds, 128
posture, 32
potatoes, benefits of, 134
processed foods, 117–118, 120
proteins, 119–120
pumpkin seeds
benefits of, 119, 128
My Brown Rice and Beans, 158
pushups
Burpees with Spiderman Pushups, 92–93
Diamond Pushups, 78–79
form, 33
Pushups with a Hip Extension, 72–73
Stability Ball Pushups to Knee Tuck, 66–67

quinoa
benefits of, 126, 136
Crunchy Quinoa Salad, 161
Quinoa Spaghetti, 165
as superfood, 136

raspberries
benefits of, 124, 136
Best Berry Yogurt Parfait, The, 153
as superfood, 136

Vegan Berry Smoothie, 146
refined foods, 117–118
Reverse Crossover Lunge to Lateral Lunge, 40–41
Reverse Lunge to High Kick, 46–47
rice. See My Brown Rice and Beans, 158
Roasted Carrots and Squash with Fresh Thyme, 187
Roasted Red Pepper Kirsch Egg Muffins, 152
Roasted Rosemary Sage Turkey Breast, 198
Roasted Turkey Avocado Salad, 162
rosemary, benefits of, 128
rowing machines, 106, 107
Rules to Live By
    accountability, 209
    living in the moment, 208
    mind-body connection, 210
    self-confidence, 209
    stress, 210

sage, benefits of, 128
salmon
    benefits of, 119, 120, 137
    Crispy Salmon Nuggets, 177
    as superfood, 137–138
saturated fat, 120
Sauteed Collard Greens with Lentils, 182
sesame seeds
    benefits of, 119, 128
    Bok Choy with Maitake Mushrooms, 188
    Ginger-Soy Dressing, 194
    Thai Ginger Sirloin Salad, 178
Shadow Boxing, 64–65
Side Plank Oblique Crunches, 69, 104
sides
    Almond-Lime Marinade, 196
    Bok Choy with Maitake Mushrooms, 188
    Cauliflower Mash, 185
    Crunchy Romaine Avocado Salad, 184
    Crunchy Stir-Fry, 192
    introduction to, 184
    Kale Salad, 185
    Roasted Carrots and Squash with Fresh Thyme, 187
    Zucchini Scallion Pancakes, 191
Single-Leg Bridges on a Medicine Ball, 50
Single Leg Deadlifts, 38
Single-Leg Squat with a Stability Ball, 54
sirloin. See Thai Ginger Sirloin Salad, 178
sleep, 32
smoothies and juices
    Avocado Berry Smoothie, 145
    Banana Chocolate Protein Smoothie, 144
    Berry Protein Blast, 145

Cleansing Green Juice, 146
    introduction to, 144
    Vegan Berry Smoothie, 146
snacks, 207
sole. See Steamed Fish in Parchment, 181
Spiderman Crawls, 97
spinach
    Spinach Egg Kirsch Muffins, 148
    Steamed Fish in Parchment, 181
    Tuna Spinach Bowl, 173
squash
    Grilled Vegetable Wrap, 159
    Roasted Carrots and Squash with Fresh Thyme, 187
squats
    form, 33
    Jump Squats, 50–51
    One-Legged Squats into Seesaws, 55
    Plié Toe Squats, 38–39
    Plié Toe Squats with Lateral Raises, 96
    Single-Leg Squat with a Stability Ball, 54
    Squat with One Dumbbell Overhead, 84–85
    Sumo Lunge to a Side Kick with a Squat Jump, 36–37
stability ball
    Hamstring Curls with a Stability Ball, 56
    Single-Leg Squat with a Stability Ball, 54
    Stability Ball Handoffs, 74–75
    Stability Ball Pike with a Knee Tuck, 94–95
    Stability Ball Pushups to Knee Tuck, 66–67
    Stability Ball Scissors, 48
stair climber machines, 107
star anise, benefits of, 126
Steamed Fish in Parchment, 181
strawberries
    Avocado Berry Smoothie, 145
    benefits of, 124, 136
    Best Berry Yogurt Parfait, The, 153
    Strawberry Vinaigrette, 195
    as superfood, 136
    Vegan Berry Smoothie, 146
string beans. See Steamed Fish in Parchment, 181
sugar, 118–119, 125
Sumo Lunge to a Side Kick with a Squat Jump, 36–37
superfoods
    avocados, 139
    beans, 124, 138
    berries, 124, 136
    broccoli, 137
    cauliflower, 138
    children and, 139
    eggs, 135–136
    kiwi, 139
    nuts, 137
    oatmeal, 139

quinoa, 136
    salmon, 137–138
    sweet potatoes, 138–139
    tomatoes, 139
    watermelon, 139
    yogurt, 135
sweet potatoes
    benefits of, 138–139
    as superfood, 138–139
    Zucchini Scallion Pancakes, 191
Swiss chard. See Quinoa Spaghetti, 165
Switch Lunges, 42–43
Switch Lunges with a Medicine Ball Overhead, 86–87

Thai Ginger Sirloin Salad, 178
tofu
    benefits of, 119
    Crunchy Lettuce Tofu Tacos, 157
tomatoes
    benefits of, 139
    Quinoa Spaghetti, 165
    as superfood, 139
    Tomato-Watermelon Salsa, 196
    Tuna Spinach Bowl, 173
    Turkey Kale Soup, 169
Tomato-Watermelon Salsa
    Crunchy Lettuce Tofu Tacos, 157
    recipe, 196
    Steamed Fish in Parchment, 181
trans fat, 120
treadmills, 106, 107
tuna
    benefits of, 119
    Tuna Spinach Bowl, 173
turkey
    Bacon, Egg, and Cheese Wrap, 151
    benefits of, 119
    Grilled Turkey Burgers, 170
    Roasted Rosemary Sage Turkey Breast, 198
    Roasted Turkey Avocado Salad, 162
    Turkey Kale Soup, 169
turmeric, benefits of, 128

upper body exercises
    Burpees with a Medicine Ball, 60–61
    Diamond Pushups, 78–79
    Five-Day Exercise Tracker, 204
    introduction to, 58
    Jumping Jacks with Lateral and Front Raises, 76–77
    Jumping Jacks with Shoulder Presses, 58–59
    Mountain Climbers with a Medicine Ball, 62–63
    Plank with Torso Rotation to T-Stand, 70–71
    Pushups with a Hip Extension, 72–73
    Shadow Boxing, 64–65

Side Plank Oblique Crunches, 69
    Stability Ball Handoffs, 74–75
    Stability Ball Pushups to Knee Tuck, 66–67
    Walking Planks, 68

Vegan Berry Smoothie, 146
VersaClimber machines, 107

Walking Planks, 68
walnuts
    benefits of, 119, 132, 137
    Crunchy Romaine Avocado Salad, 184
    Farro with Parsley and Asparagus, 166
    as superfood, 137
watercress. See Roasted Turkey Avocado Salad, 162
watermelon
    benefits of, 130, 139
    as superfood, 139
    Tomato-Watermelon Salsa, 196
Wheelbarrow Planks, 88
whole body exercises
    Around the World with a Medicine Ball, 80–81
    Burpees with Spiderman Pushups, 92–93
    Five-Day Exercise Tracker, 205
    Forward and Reverse Lunge with a Medicine Ball Overhead, 90–91
    introduction to, 80
    Medicine Ball Wood Chop to a Lateral Lunge, 89
    Platypus Walks with a Medicine Ball, 82–83
    Plié Toe Squats with Lateral Raises, 96
    Spiderman Crawls, 97
    Squat with One Dumbbell Overhead, 84–85
    Stability Ball Pike with a Knee Tuck, 94–95
    Switch Lunges with a Medicine Ball Overhead, 86–87
    Wheelbarrow Planks, 88
whole grains, benefits of, 125–126
Whole-Wheat Almond Pancakes, 154

yogurt
    Apple Cider Vinaigrette, 194
    Banana Chocolate Protein Smoothie, 144
    benefits of, 119, 125, 135
    Best Berry Yogurt Parfait, The, 153
    My Ultimate Low-Fat Hummus, 198
    Roasted Turkey Avocado Salad, 162
    as superfood, 135

zucchini
    Grilled Vegetable Wrap, 159
    Zucchini Scallion Pancakes, 191